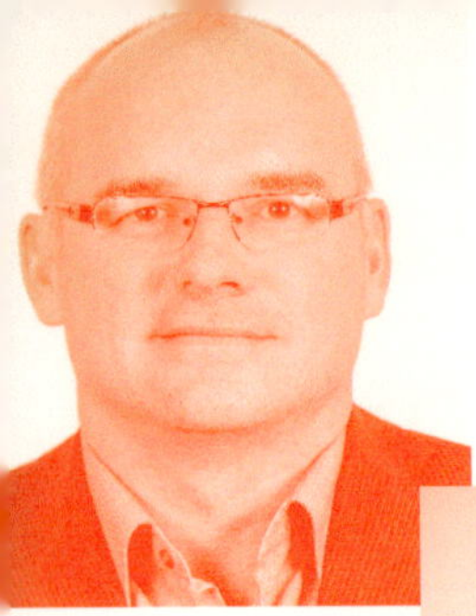
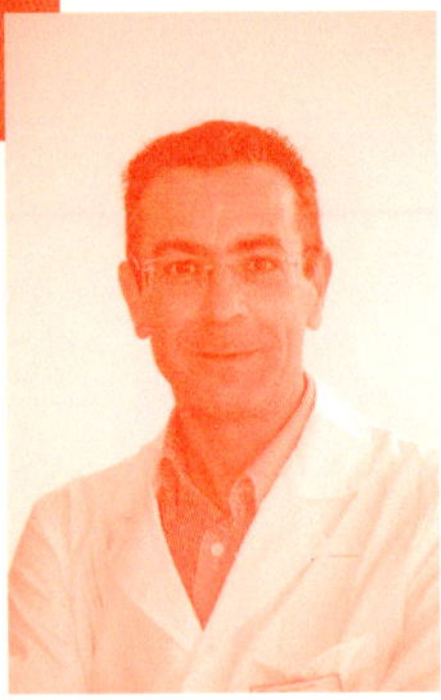
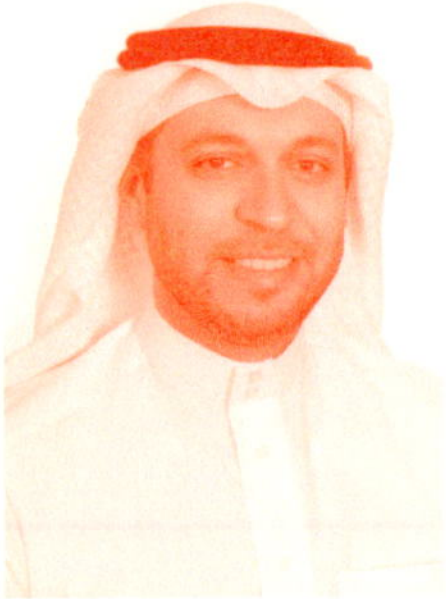
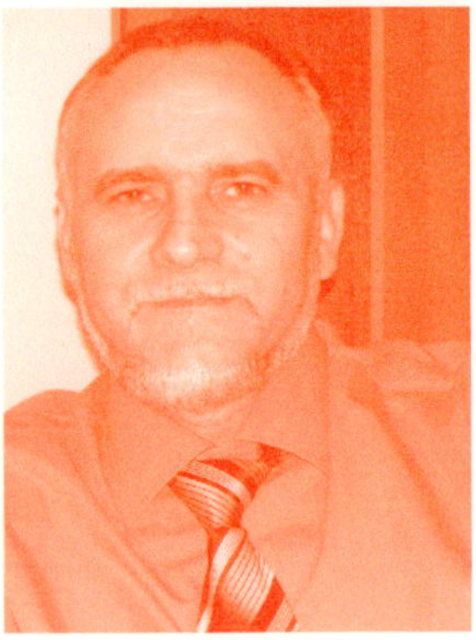
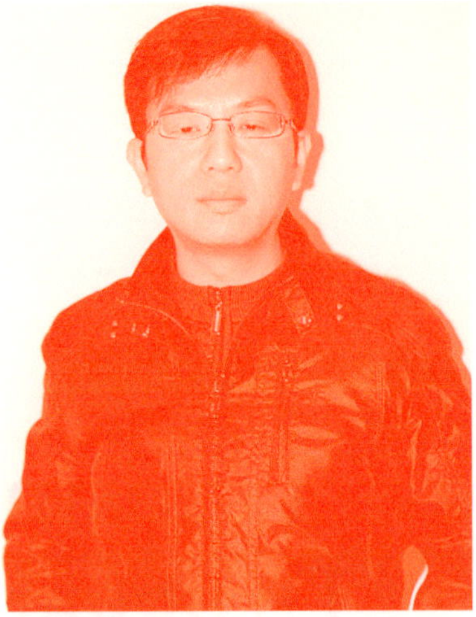
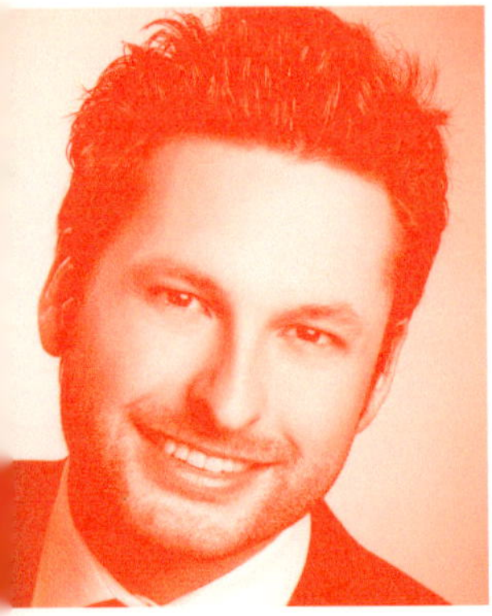
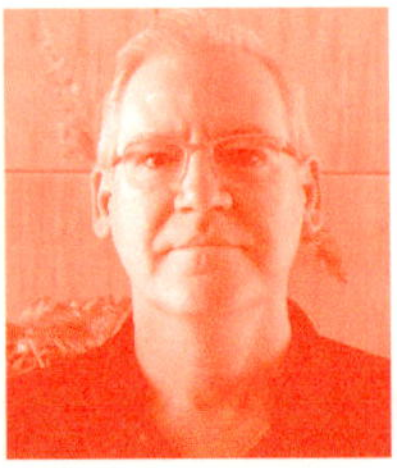

IntechOpen

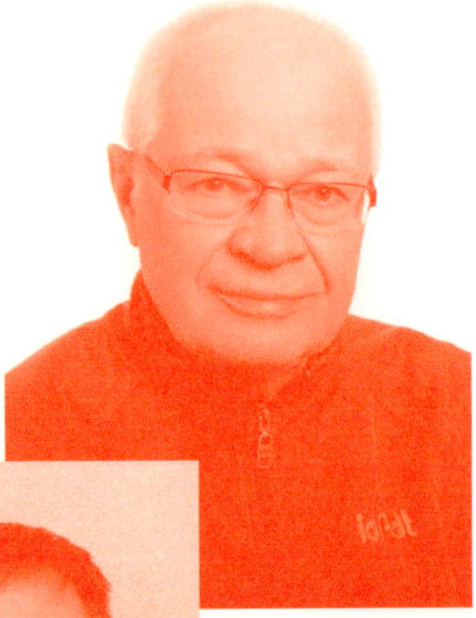
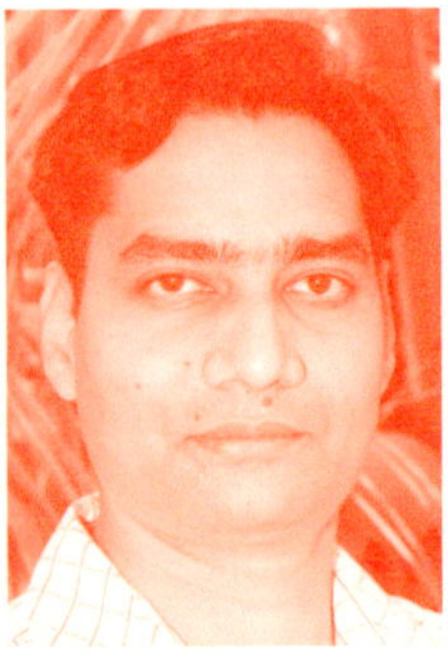
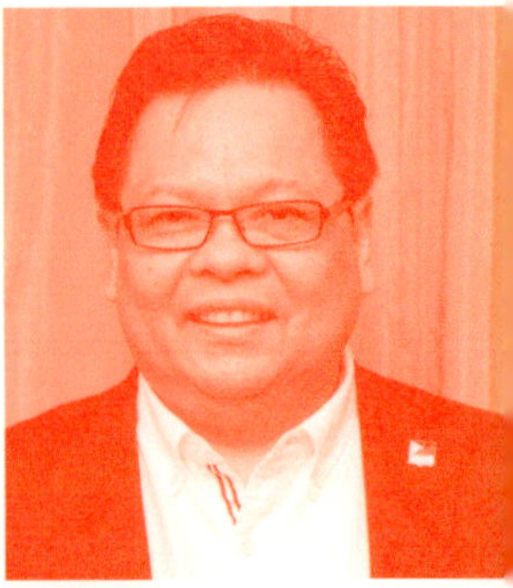
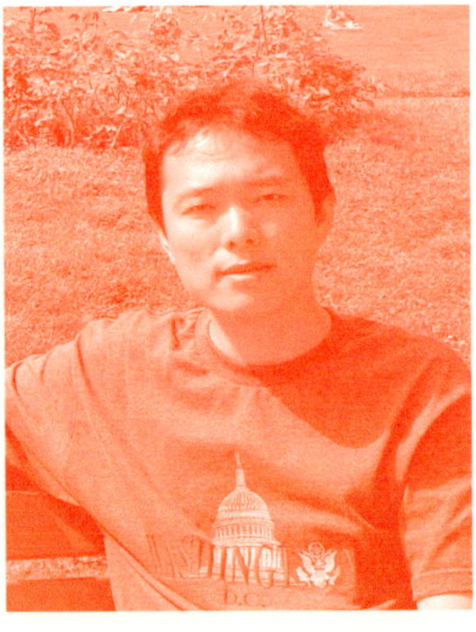
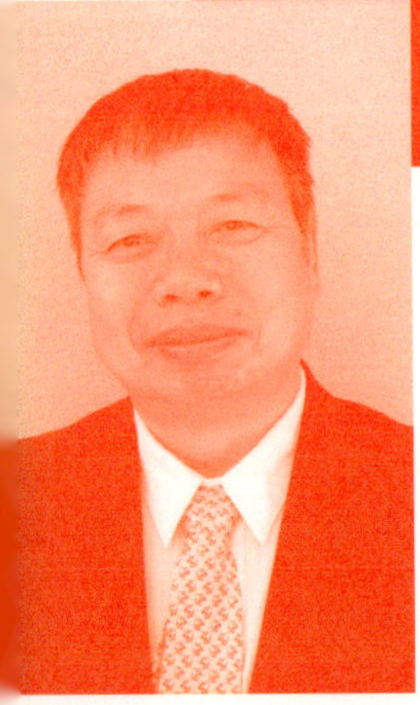
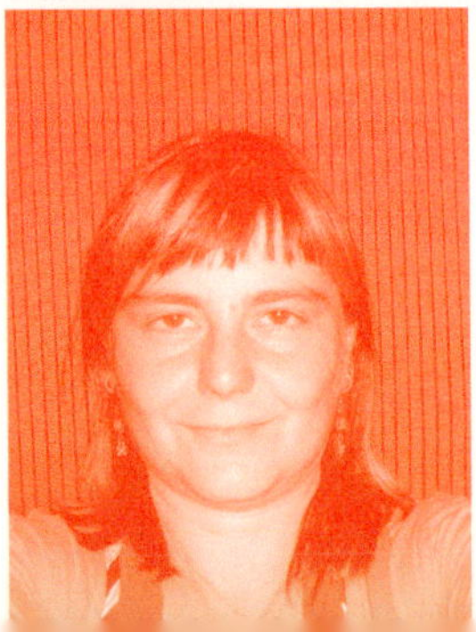

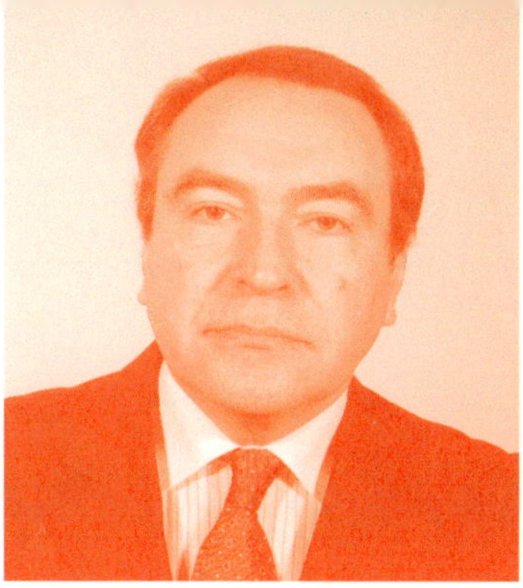
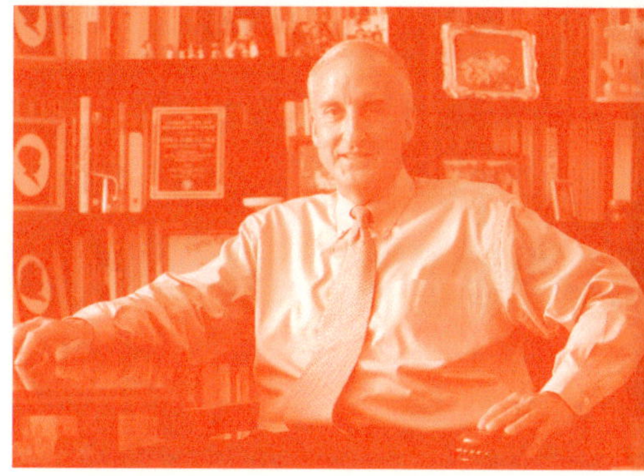
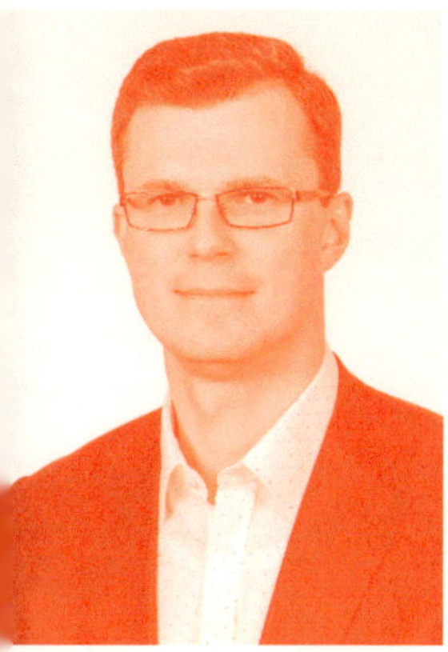
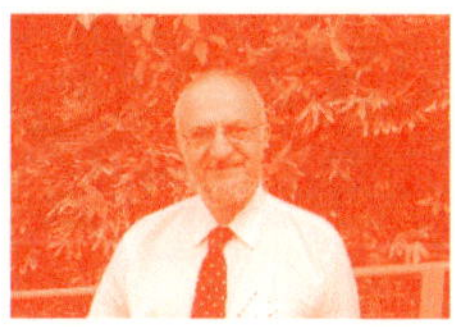
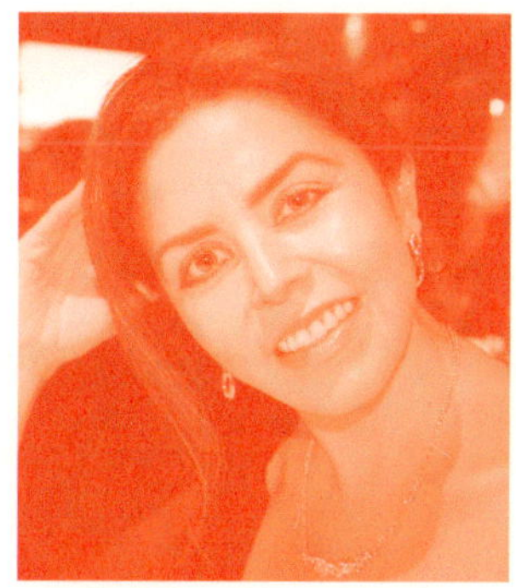

Supporting open minds since 2005

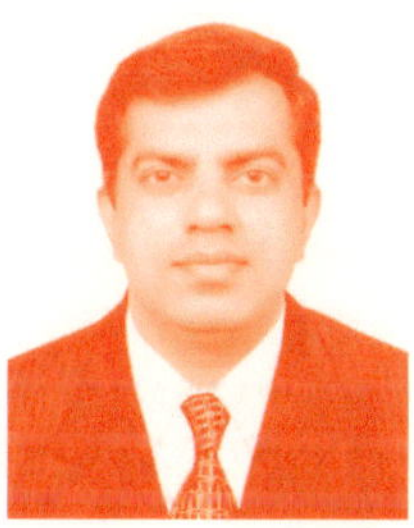
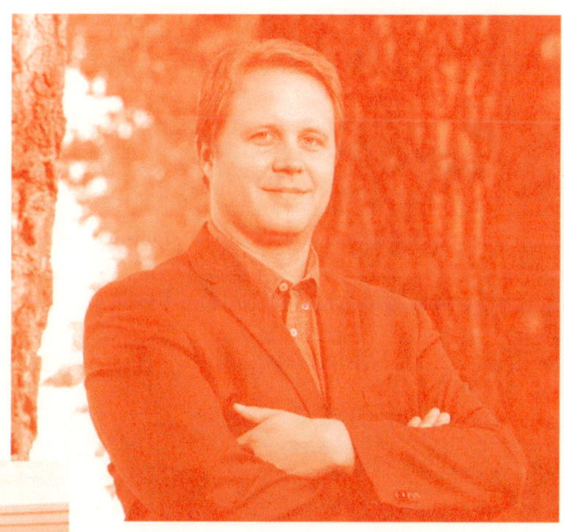
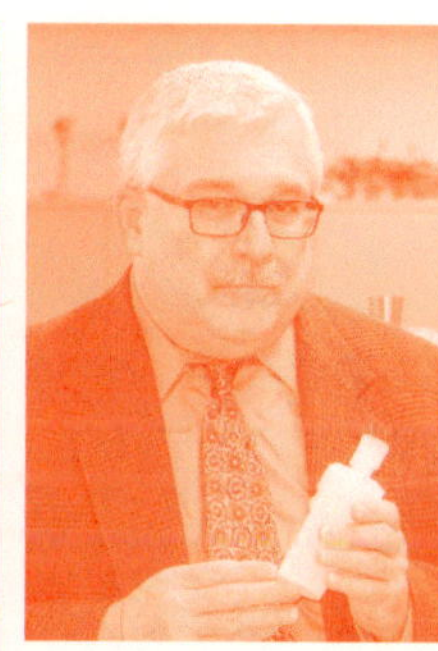
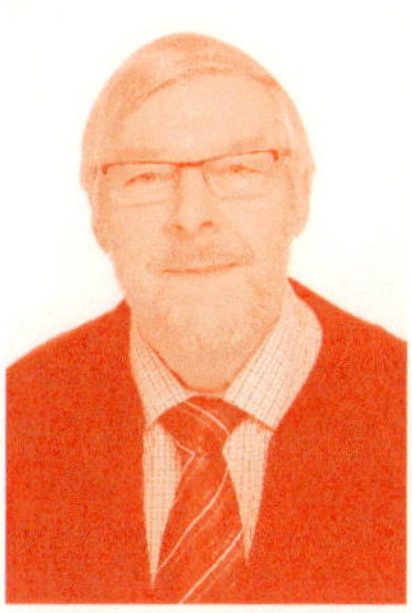
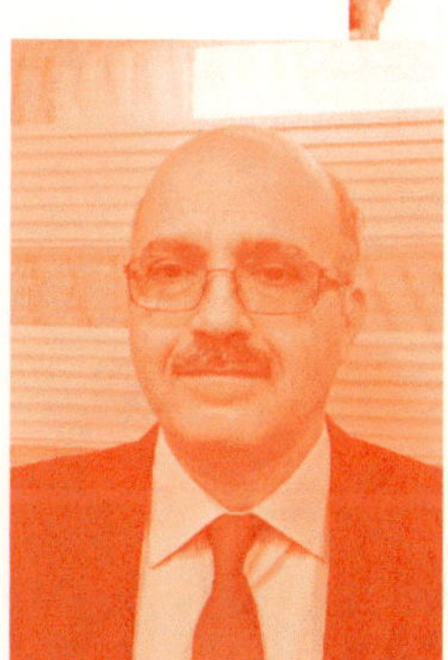
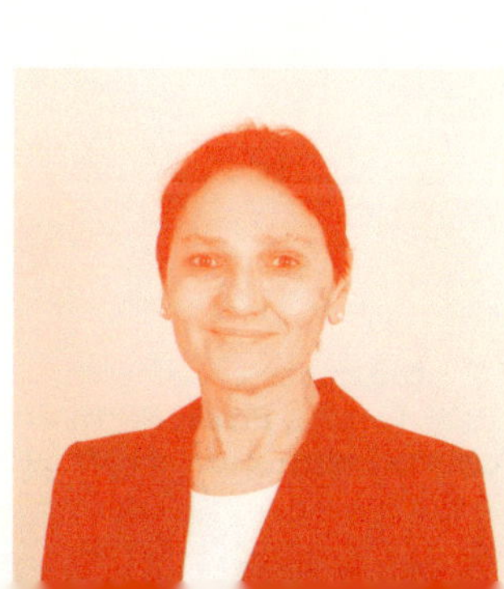
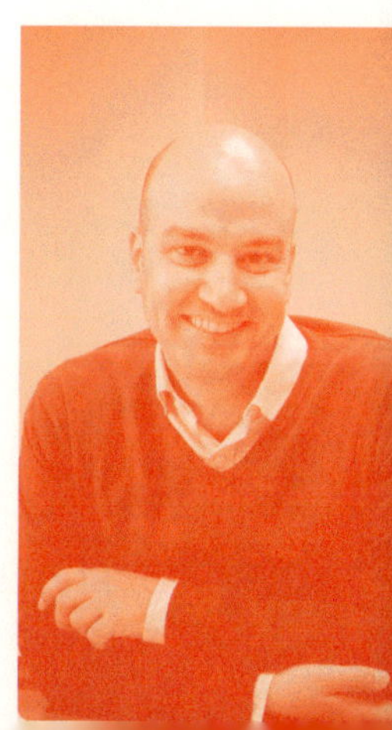

Tyrosine Kinases as Druggable Targets in Cancer
http://dx.doi.org/10.5772/intechopen.79884
Edited by Huan Ren

Contributors
Yibin Feng, Wing Tung Venice Ho, Hor Yue Tan, Ning Wang, Ondrej Slaby, Julia Kovacova, Leandro Fernández-Pérez, Carlota Recio, Haidée Aranda-Tavío, Mercedes De Mirecki-Garrido, Miguel Guerra-Rodríguez, Patricia Martín-Rodríguez, Borja Guerra, Ana Azevedo, Susana Silva, José Rueff, Huan Ren

First published in London, United Kingdom, 2019 by IntechOpen
IntechOpen is the global imprint of INTECHOPEN LIMITED, registered in England and Wales, registration number: 11086078, The Shard, 25th floor, 32 London Bridge Street
London, SE19SG - United Kingdom
Printed in Croatia

British Library Cataloguing-in-Publication Data
A catalogue record for this book is available from the British Library

Additional hard and PDF copies can be obtained from orders@intechopen.com

Tyrosine Kinases as Druggable Targets in Cancer
Edited by Huan Ren
p. cm.
Print ISBN 978-1-78984-808-3
Online ISBN 978-1-78984-809-0
eBook (PDF) ISBN 978-1-83962-219-9

For EU product safety concerns:
IN TECH d.o.o., Prolaz Marije Krucifikse Kozulić 3, 51000 Rijeka, Croatia, info@intechopen.com or visit our website at intechopen.com.

Meet the editor

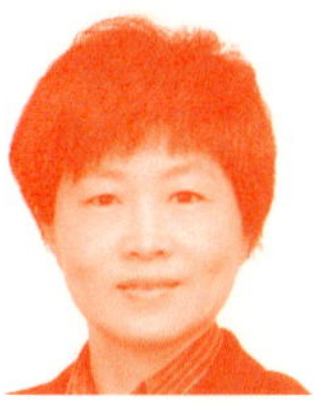

Dr. Ren Huan is Professor at the School of Medicine, Southern University of Science and Technology, China. She obtained a master's degree in Immunology from Harbin Medical University, China, and a PhD in Neuroscience from the University of Liverpool, UK. From 2006 to 2018, she served as a professor and head of the Department of Immunology at Harbin Medical University. As the principle investigator, Dr. Ren and her team have accomplished several research projects funded by the National Science Foundation of China. Their research focuses on the mechanisms and strategies of tumor microenvironmental factor-targeted immuno- and bio-therapies. Dr. Huan has published books and more than 70 peer-reviewed papers in academic journals including *Nuclear Acid Research*, *Neuro-oncology*, *Cell Death & Differentiation*, *Molecular Cancer Therapeutics, BMC Immunology*, and others.

Contents

Preface

Protein tyrosine kinases (PTKs) are a subclass of protein kinase and include receptor tyrosine kinases (RTKs) and non-receptor tyrosine kinases (nRTKs). RTKs are high-affinity cell surface receptors for many growth factors, cytokines, and hormones, such as EGFR, PDGFR, IGFR, Eph, RET, and DDR. nRTKs are cytosolic enzymes including Src, Abl, ZAP70/Syk, and JAKs. PTKs function as an "on" or "off" switch in many cellular functions, including cell growth, differentiation, adhesion, migration, apoptosis, and so on. nRTKs especially are critical components in regulating hematological functions. PTK deregulation via genetic or epigenetic changes can contribute to the growth of cancer and other diseases, and therefore PTKs are particularly important today because of their implications in cancer treatment. Up to now, numerous tyrosine kinase inhibitors (TKIs) targeting various PTKs have been generated and proven to be effective anti-cancer agents. In this book, we review a few aspects of PTKs and cancer, considering efficacy, predictive markers to therapeutic response, limitations, and future directions in TKI treatment in oncology.

As nRTKs play a key role in the development of human malignancies, hematological and otherwise, through their regulation of several vital cellular mechanisms, in their chapter, Ana Azevedo et al. summarize nRTKs of nine subfamilies, their structure, mechanisms of action, and physiopathology. They delineate the importance of JAK- STAT pathways regarding their genetic changes leading to aberrant activation, which is clinically significant mainly in Philadelphia chromosome-negative myeloproliferative neoplasms (PN-MPNs). Additionally, in a related chapter, Carlota Recio et al. discuss the complex signaling of JAK proteins in cancerous cells; various JAK aberrations implicated in myeloproliferative neoplasms, leukaemia, and lymphoma; and clinically available JAK TKIs in cancer therapy. A non-coding RNA (ncRNA) is a RNA molecule that is not translated into a protein that functions at epigenetic levels for DNA and RNA regulation. In their chapter, Ondrej Slaby and Julia Kovacova provide updated information on non-coding RNAs as predictive biomarkers of therapy response to TKIs in cancer. In the final chapter, Yibin Feng et al., presents an overall picture of TKI clinical use, and the considerations and perspectives in overcoming the limitations in cancer treatment.

In this book, we present the most up-to-date information on PTKs and TKI treatment for cancer. In this rapidly evolving field, overcoming therapeutic resistance is most challenging, and multi-targeting will direct next-generation TKIs and combination therapy as ongoing strategies.

Huan Ren
Medical School,
Southern University of Science and Technology,
Shenzhen, China

Section 1

Introduction - Tyrosine Kinases as Druggable Targets in Cancer

Chapter 1

Introductory Chapter: Tyrosine Kinases as Drug Targets in Cancer Treatment

Huan Ren

1. Introduction

A kinase is an enzyme that catalyzes the transfer of phosphate moieties from high-energy, phosphate-donating molecules (i.e., ATP) to specific substrates that include proteins, lipids, carbohydrates, and nucleotides. The protein kinases act on proteins, via phosphorylating on serine/threonine, tyrosine, or histidine residues; make up the majority of all kinases; and are the most widely studied. Together, protein kinases and phosphatases play a major role in protein and enzyme regulation as well as cellular signaling pathways [1]. More than 90 protein tyrosine kinases (PTKs) have been found in the human genome; 58 PTKs of about 20 families are receptor tyrosine kinases (RTKs), which are the high-affinity cell surface receptors for many growth factors, cytokines, and hormones including EGFR, PDGFR, IGFR, Eph, RET, and DDR; the others are non-receptor tyrosine kinases (nRTK), which are cytosolic enzymes and function in signal transduction pathways in activated immune cells [2]. Examples of nRTKs include Src, Abl, ZAP70/Syk, and JAKs and are separated into nine families. PTKs function as an "on" or "off" switch in many cellular functions; the abnormal activity of PTKs is responsible for many types of cancer development and progression [2–4].

Recent data from large-scale consortia such as the Cancer Genome Atlas (TCGA) [5] and the International Cancer Genome Consortium (ICGC) [6] have revealed many new mutations in kinases and authorized a robust delineation of the spectrum of activating kinase mutations in cancer by statistical analysis [7]. The oncogenic activation of PTKs is derived from many types of genetic and epigenetic changes, such as (1) activating point mutations, (2) chromosomal amplification, (3) chromosomal alterations such as translocations or deletions, (4) epigenetic changes, and (5) other alterations from indirect regulatory factors including activation of a kinase transcription factor, inactivating mutations of negative regulators, RNA alternative splicing, etc. [8–10]. In fact, these multiple layers of events that result in constitutive activation of PTK pathways in cancer represent important and tractable opportunities for therapeutic intervention. Tyrosine kinase inhibitors (TKIs) aiming at various PTKs have thus been generated with potent anticancer activities. It is estimated that over 10,000 patents have been documented in the USA for kinase inhibitors including tyrosine and serine/threonine kinase inhibitor drugs since 2001 [11]. Drugs have been developed to target the extracellular domain or the catalytic domain, thus inhibiting ligand-binding, receptor oligomerization [12]. Herceptin, a monoclonal antibody that is capable of binding to the extracellular domain of RTKs, has been used to treat HER2-overexpressing breast cancer [13]. Usually, the monoclonal antibodies are used for the targeted blockade of RTK,

IntechOpen

which block the extracellular domain of the receptor and inhibit the binding of a ligand. For the specific inhibition on nRTKs, however, TKIs are used to block the signaling transduction cascade either at the intra-cytosplasmatic level or directly block the nRTKs [14]. Reasonably, protein kinase inhibitor drugs target and act upon signaling pathways that have gone awry in a given cancer, whereas all traditional chemotherapy drugs work on cell division and growth mostly leading to the destruction of healthy cells as the main problems in treatment of cancer patients. In comparison, the treatment with TKIs has fewer side effects and less time for the patient in the hospital. More favorably, in many cases it is feasible to screen tumor biopsies to see if a particular patient's cancer has a mutation that can be targeted by TKI drugs [2, 12].

Up to date, the US Food and Drug Administration (FDA) has approved more than 30 kinase inhibitor drugs for cancer therapy; most of these target kinases are PTKs including ALK, BCR-Abl, BTK, c-Met, EGFR family, JAK family, MEK1/2, PDGFR α/β, RET, Src family, and VEGFR family; only B-raf and CDK family are targets of serine/ threonine kinases [11]. The aberrant PTKs promote key events during cancer development and progression including: (1) Tumor initiation and tumor transformation process. Examples of such PTKs include JAK2, ALK, IGF-1R, c-Kit, FGFR1-4, c-Met, c-Ret, c-Src, etc. (2) Formation of oncogenic kinase pathways for tumor cell survival and proliferation. The typical example is EGFR whose oncogenic alteration composite is ~45% of mutations in the PTK domain and aberrant alterations on other cytoplasmic signaling pathways such as MEK1/2, mTOR, and many other serine/threonine kinases. (3) The oncogenic kinases overexpressed in both tumors and the surrounding tissues which are essential for tumor maintenance in the host. These include VEGFR, FGFR, BDNF receptor TrkB, etc. (4) Aberrant activation leading to over-expression of RTK which is a hallmark of cancer. These aberrant RTKs are rigorously targeted in cancer, mostly growth factor receptors including EGFR, VEGFR, PDGFR, etc. Several small molecule inhibitors and monoclonal antibodies have been approved by FDA on various RTKs for cancer therapies. Presently, important TKI drugs include imatinib (targeted at PDGFR, KIT, Abl, Arg), sorafenib (targeted at Raf, VEGFR, PDGFR, Flt3, KIT), lapatinib (targeted at EGFR, ErbB2), etc. [7, 11].

However, despite encouraging results, the problems with drug resistance, toxicity, and even limited efficacy present critical challenges in both clinical and experimental oncology. Kinase inhibition induces a strong selective pressure for cells to acquire resistance to the therapy through kinase mutations [15]. Therefore, the treatment and pathological behaviors of cancer are further complicated by secondary mutations that occur in different kinases [16]. Moreover, data collected from different centers around the world are inconsistent due to complexity of patients' biopsies in temporal and spatial variations, as well as differences in data analysis and interpretation. Strategically, the next generation of inhibitor drugs is developed and applied with proposed better efficacy. Furthermore, drug combination therapies are designed and used in the treatment; some of them achieve improved results, yet others are likely biased toward validating well-designed targets, thereby limiting their capacity to prioritize novel drug targets [11]. Furthermore, many kinase inhibitors are associated with toxicities and off-target effects such as cardiotoxicity, hypertension, hypothyroidism, skin reactions, and proteinuria [17, 18]. Especially, EGFR inhibition is associated with dermatological problems, VEGFR inhibition with cardiotoxicity, and HER2 and ALK inhibition with gastric irregularities and dermatological issues, and BCR-ABL inhibition causes cytopenia, in addition to cardiotoxicity and cardiac complications [19, 20].

Kinase inhibitor drug discovery has progressed dramatically in the past decade; besides cancer treatment, kinase inhibitor drugs begin to be tested for the treatment of other diseases such as autoimmune diseases and inflammatory disorders [21]. A few kinase inhibitors are first-line drugs in cancer treatment; currently, an equilibrium which has been attained as traditional chemotherapy is still in use and in combination with target therapy. More and more molecules are selected as potential targets and developed as drug candidates; some of them are successfully applied in the clinics as imatinib, yet others are failed at some point during development [22]. Up to date, however, only a small fraction of the human kinome is being targeted, and therefore, besides protein kinases, lipid kinases and carbohydrate kinases, as well as phosphorylases and phosphatases, should be studied in analyzing the efficacy and resistance in cancer-targeted therapies. In future, an important strategy required for future development is to understand the basis of unexpected toxicities related to kinase inhibitors. Furthermore, there is a need to develop sophisticated modeling testing of chemotherapy efficacy and resistance in response to kinase inhibitors; this will help to overcome kinase resistance and allow for the systematic use of combinations of kinase inhibitors. Additionally, advanced high-throughput cell-based screening using well-defined phosphorylation readouts should be established.

Author details

Huan Ren
School of Medicine, Southern University of Science and Technology, Shenzhen, China

*Address all correspondence to: ren_huan99@qq.com

References

[1] Manning G et al. The protein kinase complement of the human genome. Science. 2002;**298**(5600):1912-1934

[2] Robinson DR, Wu YM, Lin SF. The protein tyrosine kinase family of the human genome. Oncogene. 2000;**19**(49):5548-5557

[3] Lemmon MA, Schlessinger J. Cell signaling by receptor tyrosine kinases. Cell. 2010;**141**(7):1117-1134

[4] Stefan G et al. Targeting cancer with kinase inhibitors. Journal of Clinical Investigation. 2015;**125**(5):1780-1789

[5] Lawrence MS et al. Discovery and saturation analysis of cancer genes across 21 tumour types. Nature. 2014;**505**(7484):495-501

[6] Lawrence MS et al. Mutational heterogeneity in cancer and the search for new cancer-associated genes. Nature. 2013;**499**(7457):214-218

[7] Gross S et al. Targeting cancer with kinase inhibitors. The Journal of Clinical Investigation. 2015;**125**(5):1780-1789

[8] Vucic EA et al. Translating cancer 'omics' to improved outcomes. Genome Research. 2012;**22**(2):188-195

[9] Holohan C et al. Cancer drug resistance: An evolving paradigm. Nature Reviews. Cancer. 2013;**13**(10):714-726

[10] Khorashad JS et al. BCR-ABL1 compound mutations in tyrosine kinase inhibitor-resistant CML: Frequency and clonal relationships. Blood. 2013;**121**(3):489-498

[11] Bhullar KS et al. Kinase-targeted cancer therapies: Progress, challenges and future directions. Molecular Cancer. 2018;**17**(1):48

[12] Lee JW et al. PIK3CA gene is frequently mutated in breast carcinomas and hepatocellular carcinomas. Oncogene. 2005;**24**(8):1477-1480

[13] Czech MP. PIP2 and PIP3: Complex roles at the cell surface. Cell. 2000;**100**(6):603-606

[14] Siveen KS et al. Role of non receptor tyrosine kinases in hematological malignances and its targeting by natural products. Molecular Cancer. 2018;**17**(1):31

[15] Wilson TR et al. Widespread potential for growth-factor-driven resistance to anticancer kinase inhibitors. Nature. 2012;**487**(7408):505-509

[16] Lito P, Rosen N, Solit DB. Tumor adaptation and resistance to RAF inhibitors. Nature Medicine. 2013;**19**(11):1401-1409

[17] Shah DR, Shah RR, Morganroth J. Tyrosine kinase inhibitors: Their on-target toxicities as potential indicators of efficacy. Drug Safety. 2013;**36**(6):413-426

[18] Orphanos GS, Ioannidis GN, Ardavanis AG. Cardiotoxicity induced by tyrosine kinase inhibitors. Acta Oncologica. 2009;**48**(7):964-970

[19] Mayor S. Targeting cardiovascular complications. Lancet Oncology. 2006;**7**(4):282-282

[20] Moslehi JJ, Deininger M. Tyrosine kinase inhibitor-associated cardiovascular toxicity in chronic myeloid leukemia. Journal of Clinical Oncology. 2015;**33**(35):4210-4218

[21] Lahiry P et al. Kinase mutations in human disease: Interpreting genotype-phenotype relationships. Nature Reviews. Genetics. 2010;**11**(1):60-74

[22] Montor WR, Salas A, Melo FHM. Receptor tyrosine kinases and downstream pathways as druggable targets for cancer treatment: The current arsenal of inhibitors. Molecular Cancer. 2018;**17**(1):55

Section 2

Non-receptor Tyrosine Kinases in Cancer Development and Treatment

Chapter 2

Non-receptor Tyrosine Kinases Role and Significance in Hematological Malignancies

Ana Azevedo, Susana Silva and José Rueff

Abstract

This chapter presents a review about non-receptor tyrosine kinases, their structure, mechanisms of action and physiopathology, and how they are regulated and interact with other molecules and other signaling pathways, contributing to the regulation of fundamental cellular functions such as cell division and differentiation, stress responses, apoptosis, survival, and proliferation, gene expression, immune response, inter alia. Special emphasis will be assigned to the JAK family, the processes whereby it can be mutated/regulated and aberrantly activated, clinical significance and association with hematological disease progression and malignancy, mainly in myeloproliferative neoplasms. Consideration of these mechanisms may have important implications for selection of anti-cancer targeted therapies.

Keywords: tyrosine kinase, non-receptor, JAK, mutation, driver mutations, myeloproliferative, malignancy, drug resistance

1. Introduction

The existence and homeostasis of all living multicellular organisms depend on the existence of critical links established by several complex signaling pathways forming a circuitry of regulation.

The development of the Human Genome Project was crucial for the knowledge of the protein kinase, responsible for phosphorylation of other molecules, mostly proteins which can be grouped in two main classes, tyrosine kinases and serine-threonine kinases [1].

Tyrosine kinases (TKs) are a family of more than 90 enzymes that act as fundamental mediators of all signal transduction processes, contributing to a variety of biological mechanisms in response to internal and external triggers, modulating cellular growth, differentiation, migration, metabolism, apoptosis, and survival [2, 3]. Though their activity is very well regulated in normal cells, recent studies have implicated TKs in human neoplastic disorder development and progression, including hematological malignancies [4], assuming a dominant oncoprotein status, either by acquiring transforming functions due to mutations by enhanced expression or by autocrine paracrine stimulation [2, 3]. These mechanisms of abnormal activation of TKs led to important efforts in the development of newly target-directed molecules for cancer therapy as selective TK inhibitors [2–6].

IntechOpen

Tyrosine kinases are responsible for the selective phosphorylation of tyrosine residues in specific target protein substrates, using ATP, thus allowing transmission of signals from the cellular surface to cytoplasmic proteins and the nucleus, to regulate physiological circuits [2, 3, 5]. They can be further subdivided into two groups, receptor proteins and non-receptor proteins (which will be discussed below).

Briefly, receptor tyrosine kinases (RTKs) include several families, namely, epidermal growth factor receptor (EGFR), insulin receptor (IR), fibroblast growth factor receptor (FGFR), and platelet-derived growth factor receptors (PDGFR). They function as transducers of extracellular signals to cytoplasm and contain several domains, multiple extracellular ligand binding (e.g., EGF, PDGF, etc.) sites, a cytoplasmic portion with catalytic and regulation features, and a single transmembrane hydrophobic disulfide bond that links the two other regions [1, 5]. RTKs function as cell surface receptors, being activated by ligand binding to the extracellular domain, with subsequent dimerization of receptors and transphosphorylation in the cytoplasmic domain [5]. They constitute also enzymes with kinase activity, which are associated with altered gene expression, interfering with cellular division, migration, and survival functions [3].

Non-receptor tyrosine kinases (NRTKs) are organized into nine subfamilies based on sequence similarities, primarily within the kinase domains, and are able to regulate several cellular processes, such as cellular division, proliferation and survival, gene expression, and immune response, among others [3]. The role of their deregulation, genetic alterations, and abnormal activation in the development of hematological malignancies will be covered in this review.

Novel therapeutic compounds able to target kinases have been developed for the treatment of patients with this kind of disorders.

2. Non-receptor tyrosine kinase families

Non-receptor tyrosine kinases (NRTKs) are a subgroup of tyrosine kinases, intracellular cytoplasmic proteins, or anchored to the cell membrane, which can trigger intracellular signals derived from extracellular receptor [3]. They can be classified into nine subfamilies according to sequence similarities, primarily within the kinase domains. These include ABL, FES, JAK, ACK, SYK, TEC, FAK, SRC, and CSK family of kinases, which will be presented below in this section.

Unlike RTKs, NRTKs lack receptor-like features, such as an extracellular ligand-binding domain and a transmembrane-spanning domain, exhibiting considerable structural variability (**Figure 1**). They comprise a shared kinase domain, which spans approximately 300 residues and consists of an N-terminal portion (five stranded β-sheet and one α-helix), and a large cytoplasmic C-terminal domain (mainly α-helical). Moreover, they often possess several additional signaling or protein-protein interacting domains, such as SH2, SH3, and PH domains. The ATP molecule binds between the two domains, and the tyrosine sequence of the protein substrate links with the residues of the C terminal domain [5].

The activation of NRTKs involves several complex mechanisms of heterologous protein-protein interaction to enable cellular tyrosine kinase phosphorylation, highly regulated by antagonist effects of tyrosine kinase versus phosphatases, which results in the successive activation of specific signaling pathways and messenger proteins that regulate cellular functions, such as growth, division, and apoptosis [5].

In the last few years, it has been substantiated that NRTKs can suffer two types of oncogenic mutations, namely, intragenic point mutations, duplications, or deletions and insertions, or in addition chromosomal rearrangements may occur, resulting in the fusion of genes (e.g., most famously BCR-ABL), associated with

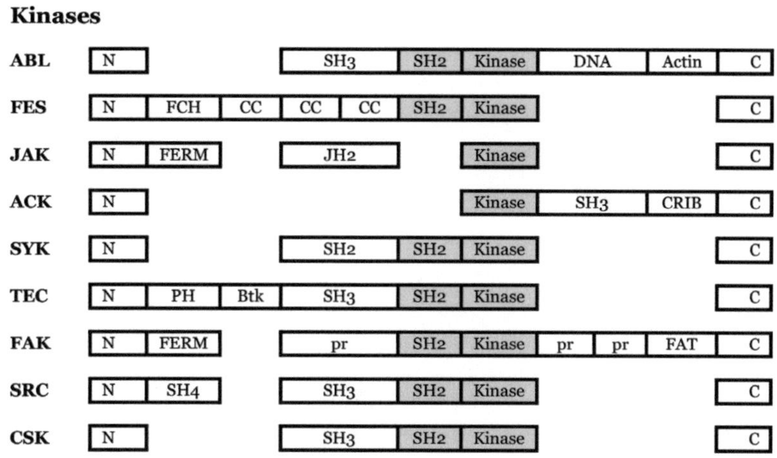

Figure 1.
Domain organization of the major non-receptor tyrosine kinase families (adapted from Siveen et al. [3]). Actin, actin-binding domain; Btk, Btk-type zinc finger motif; C, carboxy-terminus; CC, coiled coil motif; CRIB, Cdc42/Rac-interactive domain; DNA, DNA-binding domain; FAT, focal adhesion targeting domain; FCH, FES/Fer/Cdc-42 interactive protein homology domain; FERM, four-point-one, ezrin, radixin, moesin domain; JH2, Janus homology domain 2 (or pseudokinase domain); kinase, catalytic kinase domain (or SH1 domain); N, amino terminus; PH, pleckstrin homology domain; pr, proline-rich region; SH2, SRC homology 2 domain; SH3, SRC homology 3 domain; SH4, SRC homology 4 domain.

the development of hematological malignancies, either leukemia, lymphoma, or myeloma [3]. These mutations lead to aberrant kinase activation and signaling or a constitutive kinase activity, associated with the formation of oncogenes (or "driver mutations"), such as ABL, FES, SRC, and others, implicated in the process of hematopoiesis, contributing to cellular prolonged viability and survival [3]. Although some NRTK oncogenes exhibit structural, functional, and cellular localization differences, many of them share the same molecular pathways for cellular proliferation and viability regulation [3]. Later in this revision, we will focus the role of some NRTK families, mainly JAK, involved in the development of specific hematological malignancies, covering their associated genetic alterations and mutations, deregulation, and abnormal activation.

Recent advances have also been made in the development of specific kinase inhibitors and new therapies in order to target mutated kinases and inhibit their activity, showing to be very effective and remarkably well tolerated [3].

NRTKs play a crucial role in several cellular mechanisms. Some examples are the involvement of JAK family in cell signaling, through activation of signal transducers and activators of transcription (STAT); the role in cellular growth of nuclear TKs (e.g., ABL), through activation of transcription factor Rb, and of ACKs via the induction of JAK and SRC; the regulation of cell adhesion and proliferation mediated by FAK; the association of Fyn and ACKs with signal transduction pathways and of TEC families with intracellular signaling processes; and the intervention of SYK in immune response [3].

While BCR-ABL occurs exclusively in leukemia, many of the subsequently discovered tyrosine kinase fusions occur in multiple tumor types, including both liquid and solid malignancies [5].

2.1 ABL kinases

The Abelson (ABL) kinase family includes ABL1 and ABL2 (ABL-related gene, ARG) proteins, which are ubiquitously expressed and necessary for normal cellular function, encoded by ABL1 and ABL2 genes.

ABL family is involved in the regulation of several cellular mechanisms, namely, proliferation, migration, invasion and adhesion, reaction to DNA lesion and stress, and survival, through the interaction of distinct extracellular stimuli with specific signaling pathways [7]. Several growth factors, such as PDGF, EGFR, transforming growth factor β, and angiotensin subtype 1 receptors, are responsible for the activation of cytoplasmic c-ABL [8].

The identification of the fusion oncoprotein BCR-ABL1, which results from the translocation leading to the Philadelphia chromosome (Ph), by the American geneticist Janet Rowley (1925–2013) in 1972, formed by the reciprocal translocation between chromosomes 9 and 22 (t(9;22)(q34.1;q11.2)), and in 1985–1986, the knowledge of the *BCR-ABL1* transcript and its P210 fusion protein product, reinforced the role of ABL family in malignant disorders, especially hematological, such as acute myeloid leukemia (AML), chronic myeloid leukemia (CML), and acute lymphoblastic leukemia (ALL). The translocation of the breakpoint cluster region (BCR) sequences of chromosome 22 with the c-ABL tyrosine kinase of chromosome 9 gives origin to a fusion gene, responsible for the production of three oncoproteins. The BCR-ABL chimeric gene product has an enhanced tyrosine kinase activity, contributing to disease phenotype [2].

In 1996, in the era of the Human Genome Project development, these discoveries led Nicholas Lydon (b.1957), a British scientist, and Brian Druker (b. 1955), an American physician scientist, to the elaboration and therapeutic use of imatinib (a tyrosine kinase inhibitor) in CML [9].

The several products of malignant ABL fusion gene result in constitutively activated ABL kinases that can lead to cellular transformation and cancer. Activation of ABL kinases due to chromosome translocation is very rare in solid neoplasms, but usually there is overexpression, upstream oncogenic TKs or other chemokine receptors, inactivation of negative regulatory proteins, and/or oxidative stress [3].

There is a large number of signaling pathways that are activated by BCR-ABL, but those critical for BCR-ABL-dependent transformation include Gab2, Myc, CrkL, and STAT5 [3].

The first human malignancy to be associated to a specific genetic abnormality was chronic myelogenous leukemia, a clonal bone marrow stem cell malignancy, which accounts for 15–20% of adult leukemia's with a frequency of 1–2 cases per 100,000 individuals. It is more common in men and is rarely seen in children.

The formation of constitutively active chimeric BCR-ABL1 fusion oncoproteins leads to the creation of three distinct BCR-ABL variants, namely, p185, p210, and p230. The most common variant in CML is p210, in which the first exon of c-ABL has been replaced by BCR sequences, encoding either 927 or 902 amino acid, observed in hematopoietic cells of CML-stabilized patients, and in ALL and AML [3]. The p230 form is associated with acute leukemias, neutrophilic-CML, and rare cases of CML. The p185 form, containing BCR sequences from exon 1 fused to exons 2–11 of c-ABL, is found in about 20–30% of adults and about 3–5% of children with B-cell ALL [3].

BCR-ABL is the most common chromosomal translocation, but several other chromosomal abnormalities result in the expression of various fusion proteins, yet there are no activating point mutations identified in the ABL1/ABL2 genes [3].

BCR-ABL oncoprotein is the most frequent genetic defect found in adult ALL patients. Nearly 3–5% childhood and 25–40% adult cases of ALL have Philadelphia chromosome, associated with an aggressive phenotype and a worst prognosis [3].

The identification of BCR-ABL expression as the determinant leukemogenic event in CML and the use of BCR-ABL tyrosine kinase inhibitors (TKIs) since 2001 have changed the course of the disease and the management of patients, leading to a reduction in mortality rates and a consequent increase in the estimated prevalence of this disorder [10].

Imatinib mesylate, also known as STI571, was initially the standard of care for the first-line treatment of CML patients in chronic phase, due to its high long-term response rates and favorable tolerability profile compared with previous standard therapies [10]. The majority of kinase inhibitors are currently in clinical use to target BCR-ABL [11]. Imatinib is an ATP-competitive inhibitor that works by stabilizing the inactive ABL kinase domain conformation. Combining imatinib mesylate with standard chemotherapy also increases the overall long-term disease-free survival in both adults and children [3].

Approximately 15–30% (2–4% annually) of patients treated with imatinib discontinues treatment after 6 years due to resistance or intolerance, particularly in the accelerated and blast phase [10]. Nilotinib, dasatinib, bosutinib, and ponatinib are second-generation TKIs used for imatinib mesylate-resistant cases.

A literature review shows that pre-existing mutations at baseline confer a more aggressive disease phenotype and patients with advanced stages of the disease often do not respond to therapy or relapse [10].

The role played by efflux ABC transporters in resistance to TKI in CML has deserved studies indicating its possible major role in drug resistance, besides the acquisition of mutations in the fusion leading to inefficacity of the TKI [12–14].

2.2 Feline sarcoma (FES) kinases

Feline sarcoma (FES) and FES-related (FER) proteins are proteins included in another group of NRTKs, called FES kinase family. These kinases are homologous to viral oncogenes responsible for cancerous transformation, namely, feline v-FES (Feline sarcoma) and avian v-fps (Fujinami poultry sarcoma).

Fer is ubiquitously expressed, while FES is a proto-oncogene expressed mostly in myeloid hematopoietic, neuronal, epithelial, and vascular endothelial cells.

There is recent evidence that both kinases are activated in AML blasts and regulate vital functions related with internal tandem duplication containing FLT3. FES is associated with phosphorylation/activation of STAT family, with signaling proteins such as phosphatidylinositol-4,5-bisphosphate 3-kinase, mitogen-activated protein kinases, and extracellular signal-regulated kinases and with signaling of the mutated oncogenic KIT receptor [15]. It is involved in several cellular mechanisms such as migration, survival and immune response, myeloid differentiation, and angiogenesis, through interaction with multiple cell surface growth factors and cytokine receptors (e.g., IL3, IL4, and GM-CSF receptors) [3]. Fer kinase participates in cell cycle progression.

FES kinases consist of a unique amino-terminal FCH (FES/FER/CDC-42-interacting protein homology) domain, three coiled coil motifs that promote oligomerization, a central SH2 domain for protein interactions, and a kinase domain in the carboxy-terminal region. FCH domain together with the first coiled coil motif corresponds to FCH-Bin-Amphiphysin-Rvs (F-BAR) domain (**Figure 1**) [16]. Although there is no negative regulatory SH3 domain, the catalytically repressed state of FES is strongly regulated through a tight interaction between SH2 and kinase domain.

Activation of FES kinase requires active phosphorylation of Tyr713 located inside the activation loop and of Tyr 811. Hyperactivation of FES kinase is necessary for deregulated proliferation in human lymphoid malignancies, but aberrant activation is not associated with human tumors [17].

Four somatic mutations within the kinase domain of FES were identified in colorectal cancers, and Fer mutations have been associated to small-cell lung cancer [3].

2.3 JAK kinases

This family comprises four members, JAK1, JAK2, JAK3, and TYK2, originally named "just another kinase." They owe their name due to the similarity of kinase (JH1) and pseudokinase (JH2) symmetrical domains with Janus, the Roman god of two faces [18, 19]. TYK2 was the first family member to be identified by Krolewski in 1990, through libraries of complementary DNA from human T lymphocytes, while JAK1, JAK2, and JAK3 were identified using conserved motif clonation of the catalytic domain [18]. They comprise seven homologous JH domains organized into four regions: kinase (JH1), pseudokinase (JH2), FERM (four-point-one, ezrin, radixin, moesin, including the N-terminal JH7, JH6, JH5, and part of JH4), and SH2-like (JH3 and part of JH4) (**Figure 1**) [20]. The carboxy-terminal portion of these molecules includes the distinctive kinase domain (JH1) which is catalytically active and the catalytically inactive pseudokinase domain (JH2) which is felt to regulate the activity of JH1. The other amino-terminal JH domains, JH3–JH7, mediate association with receptors. FERM domain regulates the binding to the membrane-proximal part of the cytokine receptors [21].

In humans, JAK1 gene is located on chromosome 1p31.3, JAK2 gene on 9p24, JAK3 gene on 19p13.1, and TYK2 gene on 19p13.2 [9].

JAK proteins interact with different intracellular domains of cytokine receptors (discussed below) and are present in a variety of cellular subtypes. Expression is ubiquitous for JAK1, JAK2, and TYK2 but restricted to hematopoietic cells for JAK3 [9].

Many malignancies, including hematological neoplasms, are associated with deregulated activation of JAK family members, through aberrant cytokine production via autocrine/paracrine processes, point mutations within JAKs, or any other oncogene upstream of signaling cascade (discussed below).

Several studies reported various JAK mutations, mostly point mutations, occurring in all members [22–24]. *JAK2* V617F is one of the most studied mutations affecting JAK family, strongly associated with myeloproliferative neoplasms, which will be discussed in the next section of this chapter, and Hodgkin lymphoma and primary mediastinal B-cell lymphoma [3]. Other mutations have been described, such as 1) JAK1 A634D, localized in the pseudokinase domain, affecting signaling functions (STAT5), in AML, and T-cell and B-cell ALL; 2) JAK3 point mutations associated with various T-cell leukemia/lymphomas, poor prognosis and clinical outcome in juvenile myelomonocytic leukemia, and acute megakaryoblastic leukemia; 3) TYK2 kinase mutations have been reported in T-cell ALL and promote cell survival via activation of STAT1 as well BCL2 upregulation [3].

2.4 ACK kinases

ACKs also known as activated Cdc42 kinases are the fundamental components of signal transduction pathways linked to non-receptor tyrosine kinases. There are seven different types of ACKs, namely, ACK1/TNK2, ACK2, DACK, TNK1, ARK1, DPR2, and KOS1 [25].

The majority of these kinases include both N-terminal and C-terminal domains followed by a SH3 domain along with CRIB, which makes them unique NTRKs, and finally a kinase domain (**Figure 1**) [25].

ACK1 (ACK, TNK2, or activated Cdc42 kinase) is one of the most studied and well-known members of the ACKs. It is a ubiquitous 140-kDa protein located on the chromosome 3q, with the presence of multiple structural domains for its functional diversity, including cell survival, migration, growth, and proliferation, via acting as an integral cytosolic signal transducer for the array of receptor tyrosine kinases (MERTK, EGFR, PDGFR, IR, etc.) to different intracellular effectors which includes both cytosolic and nuclear, and for epigenetic negative regulation on tumor suppressors [26]. It has been linked to several forms of human cancers, including gastric, breast, ovarian, pancreatic, colorectal, head, and neck squamous cell carcinomas, osteosarcoma, hepatocellular carcinoma, and prostate cancers [26].

Mutations in ACK1/TNK2 gene are the main oncogenic cause for AML, atypical CML, and chronic myelomonocytic leukemia. TNK1 has both tumor-suppressing and oncogenic potential as it can mitigate the growth of tumor cells by downregulating Ras-Raf1-MAPK pathway, induce apoptosis through NF-κB inhibition, and activate cellular transformation and growth of neoplastic cells. TNK1 has oncogenic potential implicated in hematological carcinogenesis such as in AML and Hodgkin's lymphoma, which may open new targets for therapy [3].

2.5 SYK kinases

Spleen tyrosine kinase (SYK) is one of the important classes of soluble cytosolic NRPKs and was first cloned in porcine spleen cells, with high expression hematopoietic cells [3]. It is a 72-kDa protein, encoded by SYK gene located on chromosome 9q22 and is highest homologous to ZAP-70, formed by two highly conserved SH2 domains with N-terminal and one tyrosine kinase domain at C-terminal (**Figure 1**) [3]. Activation of SYK occurs with the intervention of C-type lectins and integrins and the downstream signaling cascade, including VAV family members, phospholipase Cγ isoforms, the regulatory subunits of phosphoinositide 3-kinases, and the SH2 domain-containing leukocyte protein family members (SLP76 and SLP65) [27].

The SYK family is important in immune response between cell receptors and intracellular signaling mechanisms, through phosphorylation of cytosolic domain of the immunoreceptor tyrosine-based activation motifs (ITAMs), resulting in the conformational changes and further activation of SYK and signal transduction to other downstream target/effector proteins [27]. Its stimulatory effect on various survival pathways/signaling molecules supports the crucial role that SYK family has in many forms of hematological malignancies [28]. On the other hand, they also have a tumor-suppressive effect in the disorders of nonimmune origin [29]. Progress can be made in the development of targeted effective therapy.

2.6 TEC kinases

TEC kinase family is the second largest subclass of the NRTKs. It includes five members, namely, Bruton's tyrosine kinase (BTK), interleukin 2-inducible T-cell kinase (ITK/EMT/TSK), tyrosine-protein kinase (RLK/TXK), bone marrow tyrosine kinase on chromosome (BMX/ETK), and tyrosine kinase expressed in hepatocellular carcinoma (TEC) [30]. Their structure is characterized by the presence of an amino-terminal (PH) that can bind phosphoinositides, enabling the interaction between phosphotyrosine-mediated and phospholipid-mediated signaling pathways, and Btk-type zinc finger (BTK) motif followed by two domains, SH3 and SH2, and a carboxy-terminal kinase domain (**Figure 1**).

TEC proteins are expressed in hematopoietic cells and involved in cellular signaling pathways of cytokine receptors, RTKs, lymphocyte surface antigens, G-protein-coupled receptors, and integrins, contributing to cellular growth and maturation of blood cells [3]. For example, it has been shown that BTK mutations are associated with B lymphocytes and other relevant cells contributing to the tumor microenvironment (e.g., dendritic cells, macrophages, myeloid-derived suppressor cells, and endothelial cells) development impairment [31, 32], increasing the need of innovative immunochemotherapies, such as BTK inhibitors (e.g., ibrutinib), which have improved disease control rates but, unfortunately, not survival [33].

BTK, ITK, and TXK are predominately expressed in bone marrow cells, whereas BMX and TEC even extend to normal somatic cells (e.g., cardiac endothelium) [3, 30]. BMX is expressed in myeloid lineage hematopoietic cells (e.g., granulocytes and monocytes), endothelial cells, and numerous types of oncologic disorders, having a preponderant role in cellular survival, differentiation and motility, and playing a key role in inflammation and cancer [30]. Furthermore, TEC is expressed in hematopoietic cells, namely, myeloid and lymphoid, B and T, lineages; is involved in the stabilization, signaling, and activation of lymphocytes [34]; and acts as a regulator of pluripotent stem cells, through the regulation of fibroblast growth factor-2 secretion, associated with tumorigenesis and hepatocellular carcinoma progression [3].

2.7 Focal adhesion kinases

FAK family includes two members, namely, the ubiquitously expressed focal adhesion kinase and the associated adhesion focal tyrosine kinase (Pyk2), which is expressed in the central nervous system and in hematopoietic cells.

FAK and Pyk2 share a domain structure that includes an N-terminal FERM domain, followed by a residue linker region, a central kinase domain, a residue proline-rich low complexity region, and a C-terminal focal adhesion targeting domain (**Figure 1**) [35].

FAKs are involved in cell propagation and adhesion and in cell to microenvironment communications [36]. They are associated with B-lymphoblastic leukemia and lymphoma cells but are usually absent in leukemias/lymphomas of T-cell origin and in myeloma [3]. These kinases are involved in regulation of cellular proliferation and migration, via response to extracellular stimuli. Interaction with growth factor leads to phosphorylation/activation of SRC kinase, which in turn is associated with various signaling pathways, and modulates proliferation and survival of tumor cells in AML and MDS patients [37]. FAK overexpression has been associated with leukemic cell migration from the marrow to the circulating compartment, drug resistance, and poor survival outcome [3].

2.8 SRC kinases

The SRC family of tyrosine kinases (SFKs) is membrane-associated NRTKs, acting as key mediators of signal transduction pathways and modulators of RTK activation, promoting mitogenesis. This class includes 11 related kinases: BLK, FGR, FYN, HCK, LCK, LYN, c-SRC, c-YES, YRK, FRK (also known as RAK) and Srm [38].

Their structure includes in the amino-terminal region a membrane-targeting myristoylated or palmitoylated SH4 domain; a specific domain of 50–70 residues different for each member of the family, trailed by SH3, SH2, and kinase domains; and a short carboxy-terminal tail with an auto-inhibitory phosphorylation site (**Figure 1**) [39, 40].

BLK, FGR, HCK, LCK, and LYN expression predominates in hematopoietic cells, whereas c-SRC, c-YES, YRK, and FYN are highly expressed ubiquitously in platelets, neurons, and some epithelial tissues; Srm is found in keratinocytes; and Frk is present primarily in the bladder, breast, brain, colon, and lymphoid cells [38, 39].

SFKs are involved in a wealth of cellular mechanisms, such as cell survival regulation, DNA synthesis and division, actin cytoskeleton rearrangements, and motility, through a major role in a variety of cellular signaling pathways activated by several RTKs (PDGF-R, EGF-R, FGF-R, IGF1-R, and CSF-R) and G-protein-coupled receptors [3]. Catalytic activity is exercised upon phosphorylation of a critical residue (Tyr419) within the activation loop and of the auto-inhibitory site Tyr530 within the carboxy-terminal tail, forming a closed auto-inhibited inactive conformation via the association of the SH2, SH3, and kinase domains by intramolecular interactions. However, these interactions could be broken by mutations or specific cellular triggers that are able to disrupt the inactive conformation of SFKs [3].

There is evidence that SFKs are involved in cancer development, by several different mechanisms. They are implicated in the regulation of cell-cell adhesion, involving different molecules, such as p120-catenin protein, a substrate of SRC; on the other hand, particularly SRC might be involved in the activation of STAT (STAT3 and STAT5) transcription factors which regulate cytokine signaling in hematopoietic cells and regulation of RAS/RAF/MEK/ERK MAPK and VEGF pathways and apoptosis molecules, having a role in the progression of CML, AML, CLL, and ALL. SFKs such as focal adhesion kinase, paxillin, and p130CAS have been implicated in monitoring of signaling pathways mediated by integrin, whose functional alterations are associated with several tumor types [3, 41]. SFKs are also associated with the development and signaling of T and B cells, particularly LCK, LYN, and FYN [39, 42–44].

Activation of SFKs due to mutation or binding to activating partners such as growth factor receptors (HER2/NWU, PDGF, EGFR, and c-kit), adaptor proteins, and other NRTKs (focal adhesion kinase and Bcr-ABL) can be detected in several cancers [45]. However, oncogenic mutations are rarely observed in the progression of hematopoietic malignancies such as leukemia and lymphomas (AML, ALL, CML, Burkitt's lymphoma, etc.), which are especially the result of constitutive activation of SFKs and amplification of anti-apoptotic and oncogenic downstream signaling pathways [41]. Moreover, there is evidence that SFKs promote cancer cell resistance to chemotherapy, radiation, and targeted RTK therapies. For example, Lyn and Hck have demonstrated upregulation and interaction with the oncogenic BCR-ABL fusion protein in specimens from patients with advanced CML and ALL who showed relapse after imatinib mesylate treatment [46, 47].

Due to the importance of SFKs in cancer development, it has been considered that inhibition of these proteins in combination with standard therapies may represent a great clinical potential in disease control [48].

2.9 C-terminal SRC kinases

C-terminal SRC kinases (CSK) and CSK-homologous kinase (CHK) are the two members included in this family of NRTKs. CSK is a 50-kDa protein ubiquitously expressed in all cells, primarily present in cytosol, with an amino-terminal SH3 domain followed by a SH2 domain and a carboxy-terminal kinase domain (**Figure 1**). CSK protein has no site for the activation loop for autophosphorylation nor a transmembrane domain or any fatty acyl modifications. However, the mobility of CSK to the membrane is a critical step in the regulation of its own activity, so that it is achieved by means of numerous scaffolding proteins (caveolin-1, paxillin, Dab2, VE-cadherin, IGF-1R, IR, LIME, and SIT1) [49].

Chk is mainly expressed in the brain, hematopoietic cells, colon tissue, and smooth muscle cells [3].

The binding of SH2-kinase and SH2–SH3 linkers to the amino-terminal lobe of the kinase domain stabilizes the active conformation. CSKs function as the major endogenous negative regulators of SFKs, as a result of CSK phosphorylation of the auto-inhibitory tyrosine residues in the SRC family kinase's C-terminal tail. Although its physiological importance is not known, several other signaling proteins such as paxillin, P2X3 receptor, c-Jun, and Lats can also serve as substrates of CSK [3].

These proteins have a critical role in the regulation of cell functions, such as growth, migration, differentiation, and immune response. Recent studies suggest that CSK can have a function as tumor suppressor through the inhibition of SFK oncogenic activity [3].

3. Myeloproliferative neoplasms and their association with non-receptor tyrosine kinase families

Myeloproliferative neoplasms (MPNs) are clonal hematopoietic malignancies resulting from the transformation of hematopoietic stem cells, leading to abnormal amplification of physiological signal transduction pathways and proliferation of one or more myeloid lineages. The *Word Health Organization (WHO) Classification of Tumours of Haematopoietic and Lymphoid Tissues* classified MPNs as chronic myeloid leukemia (CML), polycythemia vera (PV), essential thrombocythemia (ET), primary myelofibrosis (PMF) [50], chronic neutrophilic leukemia, and chronic eosinophilic leukemia not otherwise specified and MPNs unclassifiable [51]. In addition to primary (de novo), myelofibrosis can be secondary to PV (post-PV) or ET (post-ET) [52]. In the last revision of the WHO classification, in 2016, some changes were introduced, and mastocytosis ceased to be listed under the heading of MPNs [53].

Dameshek (1900–1969) was the first to conceptualize these groups of disorders, in 1951, highlighting the clinical and morphologic similarities between CML and Philadelphia-negative MPNs (PN-MPNs), namely, PV, ET, and PMF [54]. He realized that these disorders are caused by hyperproliferation in the bone marrow of more than one hematopoietic lineage, which proliferates "as a unit," and introduced the term "myeloproliferative disorders," indicating that these entities may correspond to a continuum of related syndromes. Moreover, he also postulated that the proliferative activity could be the result of a "hitherto undiscovered stimulus." However, the finding that bone marrow and peripheral blood cells from MPN patients can produce erythroid colonies in vitro without the stimulus of growth factor addition indicated the cell independent nature of these disorders [55].

But the "story" about MPNs had begun a few years before. Previously in 1845, John Hughes Bennett (1812–1875), an English pathologist working in Edinburgh, had described CML, and in 1879, a German surgeon, Gustav Heuck (1854–1940), underlined the morphological distinguishing features between PMF and CML, namely, the presence of bone marrow fibrosis, osteosclerosis, and extramedullary hematopoiesis in the former. Some years later in 1892, Louis Henri Vaquez (1860–1936), a French physician, was the first to describe PV, about a patient with marked erythrocytosis and hepatosplenomegaly, and in 1903 William Osler (1849–1919) took another step forward, distinguishing PV from both relative polycythemia and secondary polycythemia. The first description of ET is credited to Emil Epstein (1875–1951) and Alfred Goedel, two Austrian pathologists, who in 1934 published a case report of a "hemorrhagic thrombocythemia" in the absence of marked erythrocytosis.

In 1960, Peter Nowell (b. 1928) and David Hungerford (1927–1993), two American scientists working in Philadelphia, established the association between the Philadelphia (Ph) chromosome and CML [56], in contrast to PN-MPNs (PV, ET, and PMF).

Finally, the description of all four classic MPNs as clonal stem cell diseases was achieved by Philip Fialkow (1934–1996), an American physician scientist, through his studies developed between 1967 and 1981, on X chromosome inactivation patterns in women with PV, ET, PMF, and CML carrying a polymorphic variant of the X-linked glucose-6-phosphate dehydrogenase (G-6-PD) gene [9, 57–59].

To better understand the pathophysiology of these disorders, the role of tyrosine kinases in all the process is crucial to elucidate some of the underlying mechanisms.

Hematopoiesis is the process by which multipotent bone marrow-based stem cells (HSC) differentiate and mature into fully formed blood cells (namely, lymphoid, erythroid, megakaryocytes, and other myeloid cells), in response to external stimulus, such as erythropoietin (EPO), thrombopoietin (TPO), granulocyte-macrophage colony-stimulating factor (GM-CSF), other stimulating growth factors, and several interleukins. Growth factors initiate signal transduction pathways (e.g., JAK-STAT pathway), which lead to the activation of transcription factors, and elicit different outcomes depending on the combination of factors and the cellular stage of differentiation.

In a healthy adult person, approximately 10^{11}–10^{12} new blood cells are produced daily in order to maintain steady-state levels in the peripheral circulation. Besides bone marrow, in some cases and if necessary, the liver, thymus, and spleen may resume their hematopoietic function, in a process called extramedullary hematopoiesis, causing these organs to increase in size substantially.

3.1 JAK-STAT signaling pathway

Due to their essential roles as intracellular signaling effectors of hematopoietic cytokine receptor activation, the Janus kinase (JAK) family of tyrosine kinases have aroused much interest since their discovery more than 20 years ago [60].

JAK proteins (presented above) can link several intracellular domains of cytokine receptors and participate in a variety of cellular mechanisms [9].

Furthermore, a seven-member family of transcription factors named signal transducers and activators of transcription (STAT) are also involved in many cytokine signaling pathways. In 1994, Darnell and colleagues identified the first two members of the family, STAT1 and STAT2, by purification of factors linked to interferon (IFN)-stimulated genes, and the other family members were described subsequently [18]. These proteins act as transcriptional factors when they form homo- and heterodimers, among them, by phosphorylation at tyrosine residues in their SH2 domain, induced by upstream JAK proteins, activating different genes and regulating downstream the JAK/STAT signaling pathway [18].

The Janus kinase/signal transducers and activators for transcription (JAK/STAT) pathway regulate a large plethora of biological processes including cellular proliferation, differentiation, cell migration, and apoptosis [18].

All of these proteins are constitutively present in the cytoplasm without previous stimuli but can be quickly activated from the cellular membrane to the nucleus, by the binding of cytokines, growth factors, or hormones on cell surface receptors (**Table 1**) [18].

Typically, Janus kinases function through their interaction with cytokine receptors that lack intrinsic kinase activity. Cytokines initiate signaling when ligand binding occurs (e.g., EPO, TPO) to the appropriate cytokine receptor (type 1 or type 2 cytokine receptors, e.g., EPO-R, MPL), which results in juxtaposition of JAKs, and bind to their specific cellular surface receptors, inducing several important conformational changes mainly oligomerization or multimerization of their receptors. JAK anchorage to the cytoplasmic domain of the cytokine receptor and phosphorylation of a tyrosine residue in the receptor follows, creating a docking site

		Cytokine or factor
JAK family	JAK1	IL-2, IL-4, IL-6, IL-7, IL-9, IL-10, IL-11, IL-13, IL-15, IFN-α, IFN-β, IFN-γ, CT-1
	JAK2	IL-3, IL-6, IL-11, IL-12, IL-13, IFN-γ, CT-1, growth hormone, prolactin, erythropoietin
	JAK3	IL-2, IL-7, IL-9, IL-15, IL-4
	TYK2	IL-6, I-11, IL-12, IL-13, CT-1, IFN-α, IFN-β, IL-10
STAT family	STAT1	IL-2, IL-6, IL-10, IL-27, IFN-α, IFN-β, IFN-γ
	STAT2	IFN-α, IFN-β
	STAT3	IL-6, IL-10, IL-27, LIF, growth hormone
	STAT4	IL-12
	STAT5 a/b	Prolactin, growth hormone, thrombopoietin
	STAT6	IL-4, IL-13

Adapted from Becerra-Díaz et al. [18]

Table 1.
Cytokine and factor stimuli for JAK and STAT family activation.

for the recruitment and activation of cytoplasmic signal transducers and activators of transcription (STATs: STAT3 and STAT5 in the case of JAK2, which is associated with PN-MPNs and will be taken as an example), through their SH2 domain. While STAT proteins are attached to the cytokine receptor, JAK proteins undergo autophosphorylation at a tyrosine residue, detaching the STAT protein from the cytokine receptor so that the STATs form homo- and heterodimers through their SH2 domain that will translocate to the nucleus. There, they bind to the promoter region of genes via specific DNA-binding domains to promote gene transcription.

The net result of STAT3 and STAT5 activation is apoptosis inhibition and a proliferative activity [61], playing an important role in growth factor-induced myeloid differentiation. STAT3 regulates cell growth through regulation of cyclins promoting cell cycle progression, as cyclin D1, and induces Bcl-2, resulting in an anti-apoptotic signal. Moreover, STAT3 may promote cellular differentiation by upregulating the expression and enhancing the transcriptional activity of CCAAT/enhancer-binding protein alpha (C/EBPα), a key transcription factor that drives myeloid differentiation [62]. STAT3 was also shown to play an important role in megakaryopoiesis, mainly through the expansion of megakaryocytic progenitor cells.

Normal differentiation of neutrophils, promoted by G-CSF, is disturbed by expression of a dominant negative form of STAT5. It has been suggested that STAT5 may induce the survival of myeloid progenitors via transcriptional upregulation of the anti-apoptotic protein BclxL and Pim kinase, inhibiting apoptosis of megakaryocytes, and mediates cell growth through induction of cyclin D1, thereby allowing myeloid differentiation to proceed [63].

EPO is secreted by interstitial kidney cells in response to reduction in blood oxygen concentration, transported to the bone marrow where it binds its receptor, EPO-R, and transmits an intercellular signal through a receptor conformational change, which stimulates an increased production of red blood cells [64–66]. The *JAK2* FERM domain constitutively binds to the EPO-R. EPO-induced EPO-R conformational change facilitates cross-phosphorylation and activation of the JAK2 proteins [67].

The amino-terminal extracellular TPO-R domain has a similar structure to EPO-R, which is critical in ligand binding, resulting in a significant overlap between

EPO- and TPO-stimulated pathways. As in EPO signaling, TPO stimulation causes the JAK2-dependent phosphorylation of STAT3 and STAT5, activation of the MAP kinase pathway, and activation of the PI3K/Akt survival pathway indirectly and can induce transcription of the pro-survival factor BclxL through STAT5- and PI3K-dependent pathways, promoting megakaryocyte differentiation. Overall, discovery of STAT, MAP kinase, and PI3K pathway stimulation downstream of the TPO-R gave a framework to understand the considerable overlap in phenotypic response to TPO and EPO [68, 69].

JAK2 also serves as an endoplasmic reticulum chaperone for the EPO and TPO receptors, transporting them to the cell surface, and increases the total number of TPO receptors by stabilizing the mature form of the receptor, enhancing receptor recycling, and preventing receptor degradation [70]. On the other hand, nuclear JAK2 is involved in epigenetic modifications [18, 60, 71, 72].

The JAK/STAT pathway is tightly regulated and inhibited at multiple levels by several protein families—tyrosine phosphatases, suppressors of cytokine signaling (SOCS), and protein inhibitors of activated STATs [9]:

1. SOCS, most notably SOCS1 and SOCS3, and CBL interact with activated JAKs and phosphorylated receptors or mark JAK for proteasomal degradation. CIS, SOCS1, SOCS2, and SOCS3 are members of the SOCS protein family. The synthesis of SOCS is induced by activated STATs resulting in a negative feedback loop, through interaction with activated JAKs and consequent inhibition of STAT recruitment to the binding sites [73, 74].

2. Hematopoietic cells express SHP1. SHP1 belongs to the family of phosphotyrosine phosphatases (PTP); PTP dephosphorylates activated JAKs, STATs, and cytokine receptors [75].

3. Protein inhibitors of activated STATs (PIAS) interact with activated STATs, inhibit their dimerization, and prevent their binding to target DNA [72].

4. LNK sequesters JAK2 by direct binding [72].

Mutations in all four JAKs have been associated with human diseases. Inherited mutated JAK alleles lead to inactivated JAK3 and TYK2 in human immunodeficiency syndrome, while somatic mutations in JAK1, JAK2, and JAK3 result in constitutively active kinases in myeloproliferative diseases and leukemia/lymphomas [60, 72].

A qualitative difference in the signaling state of STAT proteins has been described in PN-MPNs. ET progenitors have high phosphorylation levels of STAT1 and STAT5, whereas PV progenitors have only phosphorylated STAT5. The reasons behind this and other phenotypic differences are unclear but are potentially the result of a complex interplay between acquired and inherited variations, and possibly environmental exposure, all unique to each MPN patient [76].

3.2 Philadelphia chromosome-negative myeloproliferative neoplasms (PN-MPNs)

PN-MPNs (PV, ET, and PMF) are characterized by the clonal proliferation of one or more myeloid cell lineages (erythrocytic, granulocytic, or megakaryocytic), predominantly in the bone marrow, without altering the hematopoietic stem cell hierarchy, and involving JAK-STAT pathway. There is evidence of a normal and effective maturation, resulting in increased peripheral blood erythrocytes, granulocytes, and platelet counts [77].

Among the different PN-MPN entities, there is a frequent overlap of clinical, laboratory, and morphological data. Leukocytosis with neutrophilia, excessive megakaryocytic proliferation with thrombocytosis, myelofibrosis, and splenomegaly and hepatomegaly associated with the presence of extramedullary hematopoiesis can occur in any of these diseases.

PN-MPNs are considered as rare disorders, since their combined incidence is lower than 6 per 100,000 individuals per year [78]. Among the existent registries in the European Union, PN-MPNs have an annual incidence rate per 100,000 individuals per year ranging from 0.4 to 2.8 for PV (while the literature estimated 0.68–2.6), from 0.38 to 1.7 for ET (in the literature 0.6–2.5), and from 0.1 to 1.0 for PMF [79, 80]. There are few European studies reported on MPNs' prevalence [80]. However, according to the American data published in 2014, the prevalence per 100,000 individuals of PV (44–57) and ET (38–57) was much higher than that of MF (4–6) or subgroups with MF features (post-PV MF = 0.3–0.7; post-ET MF = 0.5–1.1) [81].

These groups of disorders occur in middle- or advanced-age adults, with a medium age of diagnosis of 65–67 years for PV, 65–70 years for ET, and 67–70 years for PMF [82]. However, it can be diagnosed in younger individuals, particularly if there is a familial predisposition [83]. Some reports indicate that ET is more common in women (particularly at younger ages) and PV in men, while in PMF both genders are nearly equally affected [51, 84, 85].

As demonstrated by European and international studies [86, 87], the distinction of MPNs in three nosological entities have a relevant prognostic significance. By and large, PN-MPN patients have a reduced life expectancy compared with general population, with PMF having the lowest overall survival (5.7 years), followed by PV with 15 years survival in 65% of cases and ET with an overall survival of more than 18–20 years [78, 88].

Despite insidious clinical onset, all PN-MPNs are at risk of clonal evolution and mortality. This is generally attributed to disease progression that may end in medullary failure (myelofibrosis or ineffective hematopoiesis) or transformation into other hematologic malignancies (the most common being acute myeloid leukemia (AML) and myelodysplastic syndromes (MDS)) or the occurrence of bacterial infections and cardio- and cerebrovascular diseases, especially in younger patients [89, 90]. Fortunately, mortality due to these complications has been decreasing in the last few years [78].

3.2.1 Driver genes and other mutations

Until 2005 little was known about the etiology of PN-MPNs. The discovery of somatic mutations in Janus kinase 2 gene (*JAK2*), a member of the Janus kinase family located at chromosome 9 and first identified in 1993, was crucial. The identification of exon 14 V617F gain-of-function mutation, made by several independent groups of investigators [91–94], was one of the major genetic insights into the pathogenesis of the PN-MPNs and transformed the understanding of these disorders. It turned out to be the most important and most frequently recurring somatic mutation involved in PN-MPN pathogenesis, with the highest frequency (up to 95%) in PV, and 50–60% in ET and PMF patients (**Figure 2**) [9, 23, 55, 72, 95–99].

Although there is no gold standard and the choice of methodology is dependent on the application, quantitative real-time PCR is a useful method for detecting V617F mutation in *JAK2* gene [100].

After *JAK2* V617F discovery in the majority of PN-MPN patients, there may have been an assumption of genetic uniformity, but the fact that approximately 50% of ET and PMF patients are *JAK2* V617F negative prompted the search for other putative genes in the JAK-STAT signaling pathway that could be mutated in these patients. In 2006, Pikman and colleagues [101] identified the mutations of thrombopoietin receptor (TPO-R) in myeloproliferative leukemia (MPL) virus oncogene. Moreover, a small proportion of patients with PV are *JAK2* V617F negative when tested by sensitive allele-specific assays [102], led only 1 year later, in 2007, to the identification by Scott and colleagues of a set of *JAK2* exon 12 mutations in *JAK2* V617F-negative patients with PV [103]. Although there is no gold standard and the choice of methodology is dependent on the application, quantitative real-time PCR and high-resolution melt-curve analysis are useful methods for detecting this type of mutation in *JAK2* gene [100].

One of the most recent discoveries was made by Kralovics in 2013, with the identification of calreticulin (CALR) mutation in 73% of MPN patients who do not bear the *JAK2* or *MPL* mutation (**Figure 2**) [106]. The identification of these other driver mutations (*JAK2* exon 12, *MPL*, and *CALR*) contributed to a better clarification of the pathophysiology of these disorders, their diagnostic tools, and therapeutic management [9, 91–94, 103, 107, 108]. In the majority of PN-MPN cases, *CALR*, *MPL*, and *JAK2* mutations are mutually exclusive, although rare exceptions can occur [70, 109].

It soon became clear that this group of diseases was far more genetically heterogeneous and complex than CML. Mutations other than in those driver genes and other genetic alterations have also been described in PN-MPNs and have shown to contribute to the establishment of the WHO diagnostic criteria, prognosis, and risk stratification in PN-MPNs [9, 90, 110, 111]. The majority of those mutations fall into one of the two categories—activation of the JAK-STAT pathway (*JAK2* V617F, *JAK2* exon 12, *MPL*, *LNK*, and probably *CALR*) [112] and aberrant epigenetic modification (*TET2*, *ASXL1*, and *EZH2*) [113]. A combination of mutations in these genes and environmental factors is likely the decisive factor of the development of each one of these disorders.

3.2.2 Molecular pathophysiology

The receptors of bone marrow progenitor cells are highly sensitive to EPO (stimulates erythroblasts), TPO (induces proliferation and differentiation of

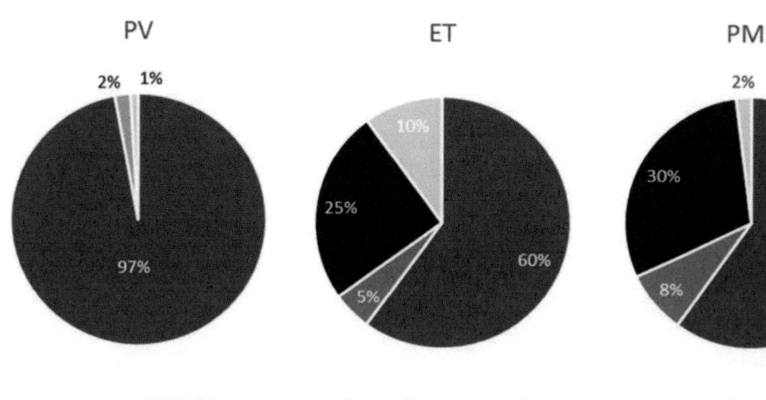

Figure 2.
Variation frequency of driver and other mutations in PN-MPNs [78, 104, 105].

megakaryocytes), stem cell factor (SCF, promotes proliferation and self-renewal of multipotent hematopoietic primordial cells), granulocyte-stimulating factor (GSF, stimulates proliferation and differentiation of granulocytes), and interleukins. Cytokine hypersensitivity leads to monoclonal stimulation of the erythropoiesis, megakaryopoiesis, and granulopoiesis.

*JAK*2 serves as the cognate tyrosine kinase for the EPO and TPO receptors and can also be used by the G-CSF receptor, all of which lack an intrinsic kinase domain [9, 70]. Moreover, JAK2 is crucial for normal hematopoiesis, as demonstrated by abnormal erythropoiesis developed in JAK2-deficient mice [114]. It includes two main domains: one is an enzymatically active kinase domain (JAK homology 1 (JH1)), and the other corresponds to a catalytically inactive pseudokinase domain (JH2), which promotes an inhibitory affect that induces the inhibition of the kinase activity of JAK2 [114–116].

The most frequent mutation associated with PN-MPNs, *JAK2* V617F, is present in myeloblasts, granulocytes, erythroblasts, and all EPO-independent erythroid colonies. It consists of a gain-of-function missense mutation with a G to T (guanine to thymidine) substitution at nucleotide 1849, in exon 14 of the *JAK2* gene, resulting in the substitution of valine with phenylalanine at codon 617 in the inhibitory JH2 domain [102]. When V617F mutation occurs, the result is an increased activity in myeloid progenitor cells, which leads to proliferation and excessive production of mature cells [114, 116–119].

JAK2 V617F activates signaling through the three main myeloid cytokine homodimeric receptors (EPO-R, MPL, and G-CSFR), which are involved in erythrocytosis, thrombocytosis, and neutrophilia, respectively. On the other hand, *CALR* or *MPL* mutants are restricted to MPL activation, explaining why *JAK2* V617F is associated with PV, ET, and PMF, whereas *CALR* and *MPL* mutants are found in ET and PMF [120].

In addition, expression of *JAK2* V617F results in constitutive activation of downstream signaling pathways including the JAK-STAT, MAPK/ERK, and phosphatidylinositol-3-kinase (PI3K/AKT) pathways [91–94] and later by interaction with p85, a regulatory subunit of PI3K, promoting proliferation and survival. Activated PI3K activates AKT, which in turn activates mammalian target of rapamycin (mTor) on Ser2448, which directly phosphorylates ribosomal p70S6 kinase (p70S6k). p70S6K and mTor are involved in angiogenesis by activation of vascular endothelial growth factor (VEGF) [61, 72]. It is known that this pathway is commonly activated in leukemia and lymphoma and is involved in inhibiting apoptosis in normal human erythroblasts. The PI3K/AKT pathway also induces the phosphorylation of BAD, a pro-apoptotic member of the Bcl2 family, via phosphorylated AKT (pAKT) and p70S6k, thus inhibiting BAD function and resulting in inhibition of apoptosis. BclxL is also activated by this pathway, resulting in inhibition of megakaryocyte apoptosis [61].

On the other hand, an increased activation of Ras-Erk signaling pathway was also demonstrated in PV patients. Ras is activated and activates Raf-1, which mediates the activation of MEK, which in turn activates extracellular signal-regulated kinase (ERK), one of members of the MAPK families. ERK phosphorylation also results in the inhibition of apoptosis, by blocking the function of BAD and activation of Bcl2. Therefore, due to the inactivation of the pro-apoptotic factor BAD and activation of BclxL and Bcl2, AKT and ERK together with *JAK2* V617F mutation suppress apoptosis and promote cellular survival, upregulating megakaryocytes and erythropoiesis [61].

In contrast to its effect on the EPO receptor, *JAK2* V617F appears to increase the quantity of immature MPL while increasing MPL degradation through ubiquitination and reducing its cell surface expression [70].

Several studies have shown that expression of *JAK2* V617F results in transformation of Ba/F3 cells, characterized by IL-3-independent growth, unlike wild-type JAK2 [91]. Due to *JAK2* V617F mutation and other mutations, hematopoietic progenitor cells can proliferate without the presence or induction by cytokines, resulting in factor-independent growth of the erythroid cell line and activation of signal transduction [102], mostly in PV homozygous cases. Yet, the presence of receptors is essential, leading to enhanced functional activity and increased sensitivity to cytokines and hematopoietic growth factors, such as interleukin 3 (IL-3), stem cell factor (SCF), granulocyte-macrophage CSF, and insulin-like growth factor-1 [23, 114, 121].

Recently, in 2017, Yao et al. demonstrated that activation of *JAK2* mutants can differentially link to selective cytokine receptors and change the signaling motifs, evidencing the molecular basis for phenotypic variants elicited by *JAK2* V617F or exon 12 mutations. On the basis of these findings, receptor-JAK2 interactions could evidence new targets of lineage-specific therapeutic tools against MPNs, which may be considered in other cancers with aberrant JAK-STAT signaling [122].

Recent data also indicate that the *JAK2V617F* allele might escape negative feedback by SOCS3 [72].

Unlike V617F where only a single codon is affected, exon 12 frameshift mutations comprise more than 40 different small deletions/duplications and substitutions of one or more amino acids between phenylalanines F533 and F547 (e.g., lysine for leucine at codon 539—K539 L), which are located in a linker between the JH2 pseudokinase and the SH2 domains [123]. However, just like *JAK2* V617F mutation, also exon 12 mutant alleles induce cytokine-independent/hypersensitive proliferation in EPO receptor (EPO-R) expressing cell lines and constitutive activation of JAK-STAT signaling [102]. The *JAK2* exon 12 mutations contribute primarily to erythroid myeloproliferation, associated with increasing levels of phosphorylated JAK2, STAT5, and Erk1/2 compared to patients with wild-type *JAK2*, and even higher activated JAK2 and ERK1/ERK2 levels than patients with the *JAK2* V617F mutation [61, 103, 124].

Although the complete cellular and molecular mechanisms involved in the pathophysiology of PN-MPNs have not yet been fully clarified [97, 107, 125–131], hyperactive JAK/STAT signaling pathway appears to be a constant, even in the presence of *CALR* mutations and the so-called "triple-negative" MPNs (nonmutated *JAK2*, *CALR*, and *MPL*), where the driver gene mutation is still unknown [55, 112].

3.3 *JAK2* mutation's role in Philadelphia chromosome-negative myeloproliferative neoplasms and other disorders

In humans, *JAK2* V617F occurs at the stem cell level and is present in hematopoietic stem cell progenitors from affected individuals, but not usually in the germline, suggesting that this mutation is acquired as a somatic disease allele in the hematopoietic compartment [102]. It is believed to be myeloid lineage specific because it is present in erythroid and granulocyte-macrophage progenitors. *JAK2* V617F is not specific for an individual PN-MPN, nor does its absence exclude MPNs. Although the prevalence of *JAK2* V617F mutation differs among PN-MPNs, one of the most challenging aspects of the study of these disorders still is the explanation of phenotypic heterogeneity and mechanism of progression of the PN-MPNs [97].

About 25–30% of patients with PV and 2–4% with ET [102, 132] are homozygous for the *JAK2* V617F allele (loss of heterozygosity) as a result of mitotic recombination and duplication of the mutant allele, promoting uniparental disomy (UPD). Uniparental disomy of chromosomal locus 9p24, including *JAK2*, had previously been detected in PV, before identification of the *JAK2* V617F allele

[102]. Mitotic recombination is more likely to occur in PV patients with mutation in exon 14 of the *JAK2* gene than in those with exon 12 mutations [133] and is an early genetic event in the development of PV, but not ET [102]. Although *JAK2* V617F homozygous subclones can be identified both in PV and ET patients, expression of a dominant homozygous subclone is almost exclusive in PV patients (~80% in PV and 50% in ET) [78, 119], originated by additional genetic or epigenetic events or, e.g., low levels of circulating erythropoietin in consequence of elevated hematocrit [119].

Although in the heterozygous state *JAK2* V617F-bearing receptors are still responsive to growth factors, in JAK2 V617F homozygosity, these receptors become autonomous with respect to growth factor [70], as referred earlier.

Almost all patients diagnosed with PV negative for *JAK2* V617F mutation are exon 12 positive (95% vs. 2–4%, respectively) [53, 103, 134–141]. Some studies have reported that Chinese PV patients have a relatively lower *JAK2* V617F mutation frequency (82%), in line with a Portuguese study [23], while the mutations in *JAK2* exon 12 are much more pervasive (13%), when compared to Westerns and other East Asians [139, 142].

Unlike *JAK2* V617F, which can be detected in any of the PN-MPNs, *JAK2* exon 12 mutations are almost exclusive of *JAK2* V617F-negative PV patients [24, 103]. PV patients who present *JAK2* exon 12 mutations, unlike those who are V617F positive, are not commonly homozygous [70, 103, 124, 138]. PV patients with the *JAK2* exon 12 mutations are usually younger than those with the *JAK2* V617F mutation and have a phenotype usually more benign than that of JAK2V617F, usually without panmyelosis [53], with normal leukocyte and platelet counts [61, 70]. Although *JAK2* V617F and exon 12 mutations express through the same C-terminal tyrosine kinase of JAK2, they originate very different phenotypic outcomes. These patients appear to be associated with a distinct syndrome, with higher hemoglobin concentrations, without concomitant leukocytosis or thrombocytosis (or minimal thrombocytosis), and isolated bone marrow erythroid hyperplasia [124], independently of the mutational variant [24, 124, 140]. The reasons for these various abnormal phenotypic readouts also remain unclear and are likely to be complex [124, 140]. The fact that exon 12 mutations are more frequently associated with erythrocytosis is consistent with their absence in ET but possible existence in PMF or AML secondary to PV [138]. However, there are exceptions as evidenced in some clinical reports [24]. Despite the phenotypical diversity, the clinical course and outcome seem overlapping between *JAK2* V617F and *JAK2* exon 12-positive patients, with convergent incidences of thrombosis, myelofibrosis, leukemia, and death [140]. There are also reports of the coexistence of *JAK2* V617F and *JAK2* exon 12 mutations as two separate clones [70, 140].

As published by Rumi and Cazzola [78], patients with the wild-type genotype for *JAK2* are extremely rare. However, a recent study [23] demonstrated a prevalence of 12.8% of patients with that genotype. This finding is consistent with the fact that the *JAK2* mutation expression alone may not be sufficient to induce the PV phenotype. However, larger studies are required to confirm this hypothesis.

Some reports have also suggested *JAK2* V617F clonal involvement of B [143, 144], T [143], and NK lymphocytes [83], also confirming the stem cell nature of *JAK2* V617F MPNs [102]. Lower frequencies of V617F mutation occur in PN-CML, chronic myelomonocytic leukemia, juvenile myelomonocytic leukemia, and rare cases of AML (megakaryocytic and in combination with other well-defined genetic abnormalities, such as BCR-ABL1) [145]. There is also evidence of association with certain solid tumors (generally non-hematological types) [51, 114, 117, 146–148]. Other mutations in the JAK2 pseudokinase domain (including point mutations involving R683) have been detected in about 20% of Down syndrome-associated and other acute lymphoblastic leukemia and AML. A number of JAK2 fusion proteins, such as TEL-JAK2, PCM1-JAK2, and BCR-JAK2, lead to activation of JAK kinase activity and have also been associated with myeloid and lymphoid leukemia or atypical CML [60, 72].

Along with other driver mutations connected with clonal expansion of hematopoietic cells, *JAK2* V617F mutation might also represent a feature of the aging hematopoietic system in individuals without a malignant disease [149, 150]. There is increasing evidence that *JAK2* V617F is relatively frequent in the aging healthy population and is presently estimated to be 0.5% [120]. These individuals usually present higher erythrocyte, platelet, and leucocyte counts and are more likely to develop a hematological cancer. Aging is generally associated with a deregulation of hematopoietic stem cells, which lose their function and become myeloid-biased and less quiescent as a consequence of intrinsic and environmental changes, with *JAK2* V617F hematopoietic stem cells having higher competitive properties in this context [120, 150].

3.3.1 Prognosis and predictive factors

Besides mutations and other molecular defects, various factors, such as gene burden and individual genetic background, may be responsible for predisposition for developing an MPN, as well as influence their heterogeneity [78, 97].

Several published data have shown the contribution and influence of *JAK2* V617F mutation allelic burden in the definition of phenotype and prognostic impact in PN-MPNs [151, 152]. *JAK2* V617F allelic burden corresponds to the ratio between mutant and wild-type *JAK2* in hematopoietic cells and is on the basis of a stronger activation of intracellular signaling pathways [153]. Between MPN patients there is a variability in the number of cells carrying the *JAK2* V617F mutation, and there is a variability in the alleles that carry the mutation.

It is recognized that the allele burden tends to be higher in PV (due to the higher number of homozygous cases) and PMF, associated with the presence of acquired UPD, with defined hematological and clinical markers indicative of a more aggressive phenotype [153]. Indeed, a lower allele burden is generally observed in ET patients [97, 119, 152, 154, 155], but when it increases, some of them transform over time to PV or PMF. Importantly, ET patients positive for the *JAK2* V617F mutation have a "PV-like" phenotype compared to ET patients without this genetic abnormality. However, patients carrying *JAK2* V617F mutation do not have a higher risk of evolution to post-PV and post-ET myelofibrosis than patients without the mutation [61].

Another possible explanation concerns the concept of a "pre-JAK2" phase in which additional somatic mutations or inherited predisposing alleles present before the mutation are responsible for the clonal hematopoiesis, determine the phenotype, influence the risk of progression to AML, and might even be responsible for generating the mutation or act synergistically [55, 61]. In fact, although *JAK2* V617F mutation is crucial to the pathogenesis of PV, ET, and PMF, the existence of the same allele in three clinically distinct entities suggests that there might be additional inherited or acquired genetic predisposition. Indeed, a familial tendency has been identified in 72 families, which is consistent with an inherited genetic predisposition to MPNs [156].

On the other hand, the role of the *JAK2* V617F mutation in the pathogenicity of the various MPNs may differ among different MPNs, involving the *JAK2* V617F mutation more often than others (e.g., ET vs. PV), which would indicate other oncogenic mutations or factors that may be determinant for certain cases other than *JAK2* V617F [97, 119, 157, 158].

Moreover, mutations in epigenetic regulators, transcription factors, and signaling components modify the course of the disease and can contribute to disease initiation and/or progression [55]. Some studies performed in mice and humans led to the "host genetic factor" concept, acting as modifiers in combination with the mutation, for instance, single nucleotide polymorphisms (SNPs) [90, 110, 111, 159, 160]. Even gender could be an independent modifier, with women having a lower allele burden than men [61].

Also, the coexistence of autonomous *JAK2* mutant and *JAK2* wild-type clonal populations in the same patient can be an explanation. It is observed that *JAK2*-positive AML patients are preceded by evolution to myelofibrosis during their disease course, in contrast to *JAK2* wild-type AML, which is preceded by chronic-phase ET and PV patients [61].

On the other hand, the role of the JAK/STAT signaling pathway in the pathogenesis of MPNs and other cancers is questionable when taking into account the example of rare families hosting germline mutations leading to weak JAK expression. The mutations induce a hereditary thrombocytosis, but hematopoiesis is polyclonal, and there is no generation of hematological malignancies or solid tumors, indicating that JAK/STAT activation alone does not drive malignant disease [147].

In PV and ET, risk factors influencing survival include older age, leukocytosis, and thrombosis. In ET, the *JAK2* V617F mutation is associated with increased risk of thrombosis, leading to inclusion into the International Prognostic Score of Thrombosis for ET-thrombosis score [90, 94, 161]. Expansion of *JAK2*-mutated allele promotes the transformation of PV and ET to secondary myelofibrosis [153]. Furthermore, the presence of two or more mutations is associated with a worse survival and predicts shortened leukemia-free survival [162].

JAK2 V617F has not been correlated to an increased risk of transformation to AML [90]; nevertheless, *JAK2* V617F-positive patients with MPN diagnosis can transform to *JAK2* V617F-negative AML [163].

The pathogenesis of thrombosis in PN-MPN patients is complex, involving clinical factors such as age, previous history of thrombotic events, obesity, hypertension, and hyperlipemia, as well increased blood cell counts (i.e., leukocytosis, erythrocytosis, and thrombocytosis), high hematocrit, and *JAK2* mutation [164]. The most important risk factor for future arterial and venous thrombosis in MPNs is the previous history of arterial and venous thrombosis, respectively [9]. The influence of the *JAK2* V617F mutational status and allele burden on the thrombotic risk has been evaluated and established in several studies among PN-MPNs [90]; however, regarding the presence of *MPL* mutation, the published results are discrepant [164]. Older (age > 60 years) patients are no longer considered "high risk," unless they have a history of thrombosis or are *JAK2*-mutated [9, 164].

In patients with ET, the frequency of thromboembolic events in different studies ranges from 10 to 30% at diagnosis and between 8 and 31% during follow-up [165], and the rate of fatal and nonfatal thrombotic events ranged from 2 to 4% patient-years, with a predominance of arterial events [164], whose risk is higher in patients with *JAK2* and *MPL* mutations [90, 166].

Risk factors for fibrotic transformation in PV include *JAK2* V617F allele burden of >50%; in ET they include advanced age and anemia, with the presence of *JAK2* V617F being associated with a lower risk of fibrotic transformation and *CALR* with a higher risk [9]. *JAK2* V617F mutational status may have prognostic significance in PV, ET, and PMF [102]. In PV, despite the phenotypic differences, the clinical course seems similar between *JAK2* V617F and *JAK2* exon 12-positive patients, with similar incidences of thrombosis, myelofibrosis, leukemia, and death [24, 140]. *JAK2/CALR* mutational status did not affect survival in ET [9]. In PMF and ET, triple-negative patients appear to have a less favorable prognosis than patients with a driver mutation (*JAK2*, *CALR*, or *MPL*), whereas patients with *CALR* mutations tend to have a better prognosis than patients with *JAK2* or *MPL* mutations.

Another important concern refers to the increased risk of generation of new non-hematological and nonmyeloid neoplasms in MPNs, with an incidence ratio of 1.2–1.4 and 3.4, respectively, compared to the general population [90, 167]. There is evidence that this risk is higher when *JAK2* V617F mutation is identified and other patient-related factors may be also present.

3.3.2 Therapy management

The discovery of the *JAK2* mutations and their relation with the subsequent activation of the JAK-STAT pathway was crucial to the understanding of the pathogenesis of PV, ET, and PMF. This knowledge has led to the development of small-molecular *JAK* inhibitors to target autoimmune disease/immunosuppression (anti-*JAK1*, *JAK3*) and MPNs and leukemia/lymphoma (anti-*JAK2*, *JAK1*), which have been tested in several clinical trials, suggesting an overall reduction in JAK-STAT signaling and pro-inflammatory cytokines [141, 168, 169]. About 10 compounds were studied for MPNs, rheumatoid arthritis, psoriasis, and inflammatory bowel disease, all of them targeting the ATP-binding site of JAKs, but none is absolutely specific for any JAK [88]. Nevertheless, ruxolitinib (a *JAK1*, *JAK2* inhibitor, trade name Jakavi®) has been approved by the Food and Drug Administration (FDA) in November 2011, for use in myelofibrosis, and tofacitinib (a *JAK1*, *JAK3* inhibitor) has been approved for use in rheumatoid arthritis. The first two randomized controlled trials (Comfort I and II) on the effect of the JAK2 inhibitor ruxolitinib versus placebo and versus the best available therapy in intermediate-2 and high-risk PMF showed a decrease in spleen size and symptom burden in the experimental arm of both studies. In Comfort I, a survival benefit was also observed in the ruxolitinib arm compared to patients on placebo [170, 171]. Although ruxolitinib was recently approved for use in hydroxyurea-resistant PV, its role in routine clinical practice remains controversial [9, 52, 95, 172, 173].

The treatment options of PMF patients are currently limited, with stem cell transplant being the current treatment of choice for genetically or clinically high-risk disease. PMF patients may benefit from *JAK2* inhibition with immediate clinical value in the management of symptoms, through directly modulating the pro-growth signals of the JAK-STAT pathway, suppression of hematopoietic progenitor cell proliferation, and from downregulating specific pro-inflammatory cytokines produced by the affected clone [70, 113].

Ruxolitinib treatment substantially alleviates symptomatic splenomegaly and constitutional symptoms and improves quality of life in a significant proportion of patients with primary or post-PV/ET myelofibrosis [88]. Surprisingly, treatment with ruxolitinib is also effective in patients without mutated *JAK2*, suggesting that other, still unknown, underlying mechanisms are responsible for the increased JAK/STAT pathway activity in PN-MPN patients. On the other hand, there is no convincing evidence of reduction in mutated allele burden, disease modification, nor progression to AML [9, 174].

The identification of *JAK2* represented a milestone for the following studies and for today's knowledge, but the ongoing discovery of other mutations in MPNs will make possible the establishment of new drug targets and prognostic biomarkers that will for certain improve clinical practice and patients' outcome. All in all, it remains to be fully clarified whether *JAK2* mutations may be considered as "driver mutations" for MPNs or if they can act as "passenger mutations" which may alternate place with the former and have "driver" functions [129].

4. Conclusions and future perspectives

Non-receptor tyrosine kinases play an important role in the development of human malignancies, including hematological and others, and of inflammatory, and autoimmune diseases, through their profound involvement in the regulation of several vital cellular mechanisms, including cell proliferation, differentiation, maturation, apoptosis, and survival.

Targeting dysregulated NRTKs may prevent the process of tumorigenesis. The screening and clinical use of tyrosine kinase inhibitors, in combination with conventional treatments, have allowed the potential of targeted-based cancer therapy using specific cancer cell molecules, which are less toxic than traditional cytotoxic chemotherapy. The establishment of effective strategies in cancer research and patient care is mandatory.

Acknowledgements

This revision included data obtained from patients and controls who generously participate to whom authors gratefully acknowledge. Appreciation and thankfulness are extended to Luísa Manso Oliveira and Inês Sousa for their expert technical assistance.

The mentioned work was supported by funding through project UID/BIM/00009/2016 (Centre for Toxicogenomics and Human Health (ToxOmics), from Fundação para a Ciência e Tecnologia (FCT), Portugal.

Conflict of interest

The authors claim no competing financial or intellectual conflicts of interest in the preparation and submission of this chapter.

Author details

Ana Azevedo[1,2]*, Susana Silva[1] and José Rueff[1]

1 Faculty of Medical Sciences, NOVA Medical School, Centre for Toxicogenomics and Human Health, Genetics, Oncology and Human Toxicology, NOVA University of Lisbon, Lisbon, Portugal

2 Department of Clinical Pathology, Hospital of São Francisco Xavier, West Lisbon Hospital Centre, Lisbon, Portugal

*Address all correspondence to: ana.azevedo@nms.unl.pt

References

[1] Lahiry P, Torkamani A, Schork NJ, Hegele RA. Kinase mutations in human disease: Interpreting genotype-phenotype relationships. Nature Reviews. Genetics. 2010;**11**:60-74

[2] Paul MK, Mukhopadhyay AK. Tyrosine kinase—Role and significance in cancer. International Journal of Medical Sciences. 2004;**1**:101-115

[3] Siveen KS, Prabhu KS, Achkar IW, Kuttikrishnan S, Shyam S, Khan AQ, et al. Role of non receptor tyrosine kinases in hematological malignances and its targeting by natural products. Molecular Cancer. 2018;**17**:31

[4] Kosior K, Lewandowska-Grygiel M, Giannopoulos K. Tyrosine kinase inhibitors in hematological malignancies. Postępy Higieny i Medycyny Doświadczalnej (Online). 2011;**65**:819-828

[5] Du Z, Lovly CM. Mechanisms of receptor tyrosine kinase activation in cancer. Molecular Cancer. 2018;**17**:58

[6] Al-Obeidi FA, Lam KS. Development of inhibitors for protein tyrosine kinases. Oncogene. 2000;**19**:5690-5701

[7] Wang J, Pendergast AM. The emerging role of ABL kinases in solid tumors. Trends Cancer. 2015;**1**:110-123

[8] Sirvent A, Benistant C, Roche S. Cytoplasmic signalling by the c-ABL tyrosine kinase in normal and cancer cells. Biology of the Cell. 2008;**100**:617-631

[9] Tefferi A. Myeloproliferative neoplasms: A decade of discoveries and treatment advances. American Journal of Hematology. 2016;**91**:50-58

[10] Azevedo AP, Reichert A, Afonso C, Alberca MD, Tavares P, Lima F. V280G mutation, potential role in imatinib resistance: First case report. Clinical Medicine Insights: Oncology. 2017;**11**:1179554917702870

[11] Lamontanara AJ, Georgeon S, Tria G, Svergun DI, Hantschel O. The SH2 domain of ABL kinases regulates kinase autophosphorylation by controlling activation loop accessibility. Nature Communications. 2014;**5**:5470

[12] Gromicho M, Rueff J, Rodrigues AS. Dynamics of expression of drug transporters: Methods for appraisal. Methods in Molecular Biology. 2016;**1395**:75-85

[13] Gromicho M, Magalhães M, Torres F, Dinis J, Fernandes AR, Rendeiro P, et al. Instability of mRNA expression signatures of drug transporters in chronic myeloid leukemia patients resistant to imatinib. Oncology Reports. 2013;**29**:741-750

[14] Gromicho M, Dinis J, Magalhães M, Fernandes AR, Tavares P, Laires A, et al. Development of imatinib and dasatinib resistance: Dynamics of expression of drug transporters ABCB1, ABCC1, ABCG2, MVP, and SLC22A1. Leukemia & Lymphoma. 2011;**52**:1980-1990

[15] Voisset E, Lopez S, Dubreuil P, De Sepulveda P. The tyrosine kinase FES is an essential effector of KITD816V proliferation signal. Blood. 2007;**110**:2593-2599

[16] Hellwig S, Miduturu CV, Kanda S, Zhang J, Filippakopoulos P, Salah E, et al. Small-molecule inhibitors of the c-FES protein-tyrosine kinase. Chemistry & Biology. 2012;**19**:529-540

[17] Condorelli F, Stec-Martyna E, Zaborowska J, Felli L, Gnemmi I, Ponassi M, et al. Role of the non-receptor tyrosine kinase FES in cancer. Current Medicinal Chemistry. 2011;**18**:2913-2920

[18] Becerra-Díaz M, Valderrama-Carvajal H, Terrazas LI. Signal transducers and activators of transcription (STAT) family members in helminth infections. International Journal of Biological Sciences. 2011;**7**:1371-1381

[19] McLornan D, Percy M, McMullin MF. JAK2 V617F: A single mutation in the myeloproliferative group of disorders. The Ulster Medical Journal. 2006;**75**:112-119

[20] Furqan M, Mukhi N, Lee B, Liu D. Dysregulation of JAK-STAT pathway in hematological malignancies and JAK inhibitors for clinical application. Biomarker Research. 2013;**1**:5

[21] Wilks AF. The JAK kinases: Not just another kinase drug discovery target. Seminars in Cell & Developmental Biology. 2008;**19**:319-328

[22] Constantinescu SN, Girardot M, Pecquet C. Mining for JAK-STAT mutations in cancer. Trends in Biochemical Sciences. 2008;**33**:122-131

[23] Azevedo AP, Silva SN, Reichert A, Lima F, Júnior E, Rueff J. Prevalence of the Janus kinase 2 Vs617F mutation in Philadelphia-negative myeloproliferative neoplasms in a Portuguese population. Biomedical Reports. 2017;**7**:370-376

[24] Pita ASA, Azevedo APDS, Reichert A, Silva CJPD, Henriques V, Mendes DS, et al. Atypical haematological presentation in a case of polycythaemia vera with a new variant mutation detected in exon 12: c.1605G>T (p.Met535Ile). Journal of Clinical Pathology. 2018;**71**:180-184

[25] Prieto-Echagüe V, Miller WT. Regulation of ACK-family nonreceptor tyrosine kinases. Journal of Signal Transduction. 2011;**2011**:742372

[26] Mahajan K, Mahajan NP. ACK1/TNK2 tyrosine kinase: Molecular signaling and evolving role in cancers. Oncogene. 2015;**34**:4162-4167

[27] Mócsai A, Ruland J, Tybulewicz VL. The SYK tyrosine kinase: A crucial player in diverse biological functions. Nature Reviews. Immunology. 2010;**10**:387-402

[28] Liu D, Mamorska-Dyga A. SYK inhibitors in clinical development for hematological malignancies. Journal of Hematology & Oncology. 2017;**10**:145

[29] Krisenko MO, Geahlen RL. Calling in SYK: SYK's dual role as a tumor promoter and tumor suppressor in cancer. Biochimica et Biophysica Acta. 2015;**1853**:254-263

[30] Qiu L, Wang F, Liu S, Chen XL. Current understanding of tyrosine kinase BMX in inflammation and its inhibitors. Burns & Trauma. 2014;**2**:121-124

[31] Mohamed AJ, Yu L, Bäckesjö CM, Vargas L, Faryal R, Aints A, et al. Bruton's tyrosine kinase (Btk): Function, regulation, and transformation with special emphasis on the PH domain. Immunological Reviews. 2009;**228**:58-73

[32] Mohammad DK, Nore BF, Hussain A, Gustafsson MO, Mohamed AJ, Smith CI. Dual phosphorylation of Btk by Akt/protein kinase b provides docking for 14-3-3ζ, regulates shuttling, and attenuates both tonic and induced signaling in B cells. Molecular and Cellular Biology. 2013;**33**:3214-3226

[33] Tojo A. Kinase inhibitors against hematological malignancies. Nihon Rinsho. 2014;**72**:1118-1124

[34] Yu L, Simonson OE, Mohamed AJ, Smith CI. NF-kappaB regulates

the transcription of protein tyrosine kinase TEC. The FEBS Journal. 2009;**276**:6714-6724

[35] Lietha D, Cai X, Ceccarelli DF, Li Y, Schaller MD, Eck MJ. Structural basis for the autoinhibition of focal adhesion kinase. Cell. 2007;**129**:1177-1187

[36] Yin B. Focal adhesion kinase as a target in the treatment of hematological malignancies. Leukemia Research. 2011;**35**:1416-1418

[37] Carter BZ, Mak PY, Wang X, Yang H, Garcia-Manero G, Mak DH, et al. Focal adhesion kinase as a potential target in AML and MDS. Molecular Cancer Therapeutics. 2017;**16**:1133-1144

[38] Sen B, Johnson FM. Regulation of SRC family kinases in human cancers. Journal of Signal Transduction. 2011;**2011**:865819

[39] Parsons SJ, Parsons JT. SRC family kinases, key regulators of signal transduction. Oncogene. 2004;**23**:7906-7909

[40] Boggon TJ, Eck MJ. Structure and regulation of SRC family kinases. Oncogene. 2004;**23**:7918-7927

[41] Ku M, Wall M, MacKinnon RN, Walkley CR, Purton LE, Tam C, et al. SRC family kinases and their role in hematological malignancies. Leukemia & Lymphoma. 2015;**56**:577-586

[42] Palacios EH, Weiss A. Function of the SRC-family kinases, Lck and Fyn, in T-cell development and activation. Oncogene. 2004;**23**:7990-8000

[43] Salmond RJ, Filby A, Qureshi I, Caserta S, Zamoyska R. T-cell receptor proximal signaling via the SRC-family kinases, Lck and Fyn, influences T-cell activation, differentiation, and tolerance. Immunological Reviews. 2009;**228**:9-22

[44] Elias D, Ditzel HJ. Fyn is an important molecule in cancer pathogenesis and drug resistance. Pharmacological Research. 2015;**100**:250-254

[45] Kim MS, Kim GM, Choi YJ, Kim HJ, Kim YJ, Jin W. c-SRC activation through a TrkA and c-SRC interaction is essential for cell proliferation and hematological malignancies. Biochemical and Biophysical Research Communications. 2013;**441**:431-437

[46] Warmuth M, Damoiseaux R, Liu Y, Fabbro D, Gray N. SRC family kinases: Potential targets for the treatment of human cancer and leukemia. Current Pharmaceutical Design. 2003;**9**:2043-2059

[47] Pene-Dumitrescu T, Smithgall TE. Expression of a SRC family kinase in chronic myelogenous leukemia cells induces resistance to imatinib in a kinase-dependent manner. The Journal of Biological Chemistry. 2010;**285**:21446-21457

[48] Zhang S, Yu D. Targeting SRC family kinases in anti-cancer therapies: Turning promise into triumph. Trends in Pharmacological Sciences. 2012;**33**:122-128

[49] Okada M. Regulation of the SRC family kinases by CSK. International Journal of Biological Sciences. 2012;**8**:1385-1397

[50] Vardiman JW, Harris NL, Brunning RD. The World Health Organization (WHO) classification of the myeloid neoplasms. Blood. 2002;**100**:2292-2302

[51] Swerdlow SH, Campo E, Harris NL, Jaffe ES, Pileri SA, Stein H, et al. WHO Classification of Tumours of Haematopioetic and Lymphoid Tissues. Lyon: World Health Organization; 2008

[52] Tefferi A, Barbui T. Polycythemia vera and essential thrombocythemia: 2017 update on diagnosis, risk-stratification, and management. American Journal of Hematology. 2017;**92**:94-108

[53] Arber DA, Orazi A, Hasserjian R, Thiele J, Borowitz MJ, Le Beau MM, et al. The 2016 revision to the World Health Organization classification of myeloid neoplasms and acute leukemia. Blood. 2016;**127**:2391-2405

[54] DAMESHEK W. Some speculations on the myeloproliferative syndromes. Blood. 1951;**6**:372-375

[55] Skoda RC, Duek A, Grisouard J. Pathogenesis of myeloproliferative neoplasms. Experimental Hematology. 2015;**43**:599-608

[56] NOWELL PC, HUNGERFORD DA. Chromosome studies on normal and leukemic human leukocytes. Journal of the National Cancer Institute. 1960;**25**:85-109

[57] Adamson JW, Fialkow PJ, Murphy S, Prchal JF, Steinmann L. Polycythemia vera: Stem-cell and probable clonal origin of the disease. The New England Journal of Medicine. 1976;**295**:913-916

[58] Fialkow PJ. Glucose-6-phosphate dehydrogenase (G-6-PD) markers in Burkitt lymphoma and other malignancies. Haematology and Blood Transfusion. 1977;**20**:297-305

[59] Fialkow PJ, Faguet GB, Jacobson RJ, Vaidya K, Murphy S. Evidence that essential thrombocythemia is a clonal disorder with origin in a multipotent stem cell. Blood. 1981;**58**:916-919

[60] Babon JJ, Lucet IS, Murphy JM, Nicola NA, Varghese LN. The molecular regulation of Janus kinase (JAK) activation. Biochemical Journal. 2014;**462**:1-13

[61] Koopmans SM, Schouten HC, van Marion AM. BCR-ABL negative myeloproliferative neoplasia: A review of involved molecular mechanisms. Histology and Histopathology. 2015;**30**:151-161

[62] Numata A, Shimoda K, Kamezaki K, Haro T, Kakumitsu H, Shide K, et al. Signal transducers and activators of transcription 3 augments the transcriptional activity of CCAAT/enhancer-binding protein alpha in granulocyte colony-stimulating factor signaling pathway. The Journal of Biological Chemistry. 2005;**280**:12621-12629

[63] Kieslinger M, Woldman I, Moriggl R, Hofmann J, Marine JC, Ihle JN, et al. Antiapoptotic activity of Stat5 required during terminal stages of myeloid differentiation. Genes & Development. 2000;**14**:232-244

[64] Jacobson LO, Goldwasser E, Fried W, Plzak L. Role of the kidney in erythropoiesis. Nature. 1957;**179**:633-634

[65] Maxwell AP, Lappin TR, Johnston CF, Bridges JM, McGeown MG. Erythropoietin production in kidney tubular cells. British Journal of Haematology. 1990;**74**:535-539

[66] Remy I, Wilson IA, Michnick SW. Erythropoietin receptor activation by a ligand-induced conformation change. Science. 1999;**283**:990-993

[67] Witthuhn BA, Quelle FW, Silvennoinen O, Yi T, Tang B, Miura O, et al. JAK2 associates with the erythropoietin receptor and is tyrosine phosphorylated and activated following stimulation with erythropoietin. Cell. 1993;**74**:227-236

[68] Kralovics R, Buser AS, Teo SS, Coers J, Tichelli A, van der Maas AP,

et al. Comparison of molecular markers in a cohort of patients with chronic myeloproliferative disorders. Blood. 2003;**102**:1869-1871

[69] Li Y, Hetet G, Maurer AM, Chait Y, Dhermy D, Briere J. Spontaneous megakaryocyte colony formation in myeloproliferative disorders is not neutralizable by antibodies against IL3, IL6 and GM-CSF. British Journal of Haematology. 1994;**87**:471-476

[70] Spivak JL. Myeloproliferative Neoplasms. The New England Journal of Medicine. 2017;**376**:2168-2181

[71] Levine RL, Pardanani A, Tefferi A, Gilliland DG. Role of JAK2 in the pathogenesis and therapy of myeloproliferative disorders. Nature Reviews. Cancer. 2007;7:673-683

[72] Meyer SC, Levine RL. Molecular pathways: Molecular basis for sensitivity and resistance to JAK kinase inhibitors. Clinical Cancer Research. 2014;**20**:2051-2059

[73] Rawlings JS, Rosler KM, Harrison DA. The JAK/STAT signaling pathway. Journal of Cell Science. 2004;**117**:1281-1283

[74] Espert L, Dusanter-Fourt I, Chelbi-Alix MK. Negative regulation of the JAK/STAT: Pathway implication in tumorigenesis. Bulletin du Cancer. 2005;**92**:845-857

[75] Valentino L, Pierre J. JAK/STAT signal transduction: Regulators and implication in hematological malignancies. Biochemical Pharmacology. 2006;**71**:713-721

[76] Jones AV, Cross NC. Inherited predisposition to myeloproliferative neoplasms. Therapeutic Advances in Hematology. 2013;**4**:237-253

[77] Passamonti F, Mora B, Maffioli M. New molecular genetics in the diagnosis and treatment of myeloproliferative neoplasms. Current Opinion in Hematology. 2016;**23**:137-143

[78] Rumi E, Cazzola M. Diagnosis, risk stratification, and response evaluation in classical myeloproliferative neoplasms. Blood. 2017;**129**:680-692

[79] Titmarsh GJ, Duncombe AS, McMullin MF, O'Rorke M, Mesa R, De Vocht F, et al. How common are myeloproliferative neoplasms? A systematic review and meta-analysis. American Journal of Hematology. 2014;**89**:581-587

[80] Moulard O, Mehta J, Fryzek J, Olivares R, Iqbal U, Mesa RA. Epidemiology of myelofibrosis, essential thrombocythemia, and polycythemia vera in the European Union. European Journal of Haematology. 2014;**92**:289-297

[81] Mehta J, Wang H, Iqbal SU, Mesa R. Epidemiology of myeloproliferative neoplasms in the United States. Leukemia & Lymphoma. 2014;**55**:595-600

[82] Srour SA, Devesa SS, Morton LM, Check DP, Curtis RE, Linet MS, et al. Incidence and patient survival of myeloproliferative neoplasms and myelodysplastic/myeloproliferative neoplasms in the United States, 2001-12. British Journal of Haematology. 2016;**174**:382-396

[83] Bellanné-Chantelot C, Chaumarel I, Labopin M, Bellanger F, Barbu V, De Toma C, et al. Genetic and clinical implications of the Val617Phe JAK2 mutation in 72 families with myeloproliferative disorders. Blood. 2006;**108**:346-352

[84] Passamonti F, Rumi E, Arcaini L, Boveri E, Elena C, Pietra D, et al. Prognostic factors for thrombosis, myelofibrosis, and leukemia in essential thrombocythemia: A study

of 605 patients. Haematologica. 2008;**93**:1645-1651

[85] Bai J, Xue Y, Ye L, Yao J, Zhou C, Shao Z, et al. Risk factors of long-term incidences of thrombosis, myelofibrosis and evolution into malignance in polycythemia vera: A single center experience from China. International Journal of Hematology. 2008;**88**:530-535

[86] Hultcrantz M, Kristinsson SY, Andersson TM, Landgren O, Eloranta S, Derolf AR, et al. Patterns of survival among patients with myeloproliferative neoplasms diagnosed in Sweden from 1973 to 2008: A population-based study. Journal of Clinical Oncology. 2012;**30**:2995-3001

[87] Tefferi A, Guglielmelli P, Larson DR, Finke C, Wassie EA, Pieri L, et al. Long-term survival and blast transformation in molecularly annotated essential thrombocythemia, polycythemia vera, and myelofibrosis. Blood. 2014;**124**:2507-2513 (quiz 2615)

[88] Tefferi A. Essential thrombocythemia, polycythemia vera, and myelofibrosis: Current management and the prospect of targeted therapy. American Journal of Hematology. 2008;**83**:491-497

[89] Hultcrantz M, Wilkes SR, Kristinsson SY, Andersson TM, Derolf Å, Eloranta S, et al. Risk and cause of death in patients diagnosed with myeloproliferative neoplasms in sweden between 1973 and 2005: A population-based study. Journal of Clinical Oncology. 2015;**33**:2288-2295

[90] Azevedo AP, Silva SN, Reichert A, Lima F, Júnior E, Rueff J. Effects of polymorphic DNA genes involved in BER and caspase pathways on the clinical outcome of myeloproliferative neoplasms under treatment with hydroxyurea. Molecular Medicine Reports. 2018;**18**:5243-5255

[91] James C, Ugo V, Le Couédic JP, Staerk J, Delhommeau F, Lacout C, et al. A unique clonal JAK2 mutation leading to constitutive signalling causes polycythaemia vera. Nature. 2005;**434**:1144-1148

[92] Kralovics R, Passamonti F, Buser AS, Teo SS, Tiedt R, Passweg JR, et al. A gain-of-function mutation of JAK2 in myeloproliferative disorders. The New England Journal of Medicine. 2005;**352**:1779-1790

[93] Levine RL, Wadleigh M, Cools J, Ebert BL, Wernig G, Huntly BJ, et al. Activating mutation in the tyrosine kinase JAK2 in polycythemia vera, essential thrombocythemia, and myeloid metaplasia with myelofibrosis. Cancer Cell. 2005;**7**:387-397

[94] Baxter EJ, Scott LM, Campbell PJ, East C, Fourouclas N, Swanton S, et al. Acquired mutation of the tyrosine kinase JAK2 in human myeloproliferative disorders. Lancet. 2005;**365**:1054-1061

[95] Tefferi A, Pardanani A. Myeloproliferative neoplasms: A contemporary review. JAMA Osncology. 2015;**1**:97-105

[96] Levine RL. Mechanisms of mutations in myeloproliferative neoplasms. Best Practice & Research. Clinical Haematology. 2009;**22**:489-494

[97] Hinds DA, Barnholt KE, Mesa RA, Kiefer AK, Do CB, Eriksson N, et al. Germ line variants predispose to both JAK2 V617F clonal hematopoiesis and myeloproliferative neoplasms. Blood. 2016;**128**:1121-1128

[98] Cazzola M, Kralovics R. From Janus kinase 2 to calreticulin: The clinically relevant genomic landscape of myeloproliferative neoplasms. Blood. 2014;**123**:3714-3719

[99] Oh ST, Gotlib J. JAK2 V617F and beyond: Role of genetics and aberrant signaling in the pathogenesis of myeloproliferative neoplasms. Expert Review of Hematology. 2010;**3**:323-337

[100] Bench AJ, Baxter EJ, Green AR. Methods for detecting mutations in the human JAK2 gene. Methods in Molecular Biology. 2013;**967**:115-131

[101] Pikman Y, Lee BH, Mercher T, McDowell E, Ebert BL, Gozo M, et al. MPLW515L is a novel somatic activating mutation in myelofibrosis with myeloid metaplasia. PLoS Medicine. 2006;**3**:e270

[102] Tefferi A. JAK and MPL mutations in myeloid malignancies. Leukemia & Lymphoma. 2008;**49**:388-397

[103] Scott LM, Tong W, Levine RL, Scott MA, Beer PA, Stratton MR, et al. JAK2 exon 12 mutations in polycythemia vera and idiopathic erythrocytosis. The New England Journal of Medicine. 2007;**356**:459-468

[104] Nangalia J, Green TR. The evolving genomic landscape of myeloproliferative neoplasms. Hematology. American Society of Hematology. Education Program. 2014;**2014**:287-296

[105] Langabeer SE, Andrikovics H, Asp J, Bellosillo B, Carillo S, Haslam K, et al. MPN&MPNr-EuroNet, molecular diagnostics of myeloproliferative neoplasms. European Journal of Haematology. 2015;**95**:270-279

[106] Klampfl T, Gisslinger H, Harutyunyan AS, Nivarthi H, Rumi E, Milosevic JD, et al. Somatic mutations of calreticulin in myeloproliferative neoplasms. The New England Journal of Medicine. 2013;**369**:2379-2390

[107] Delhommeau F, Jeziorowska D, Marzac C, Casadevall N. Molecular aspects of myeloproliferative neoplasms. International Journal of Hematology. 2010;**91**:165-173

[108] Mambet C, Matei L, Necula LG, Diaconu CC. A link between the driver mutations and dysregulated apoptosis in BCR-ABL1 negative myeloproliferative neoplasms. Journal of Immunoassay & Immunochemistry. 2016;**37**:331-345

[109] Kang MG, Choi HW, Lee JH, Choi YJ, Choi HJ, Shin JH, et al. Coexistence of JAK2 and CALR mutations and their clinical implications in patients with essential thrombocythemia. Oncotarget. 2016;7:57036-57049

[110] Azevedo AP, Silva SN, De Lima JP, Reichert A, Lima F, Júnior E, et al. DNA repair genes polymorphisms and genetic susceptibility to Philadelphia-negative myeloproliferative neoplasms in a Portuguese population: The role of base excision repair genes polymorphisms. Oncology Letters. 2017;**13**:4641-4650

[111] Azevedo AP, Silva S, Reichert A, Lima F, Júnior E, Rueff J. The role of caspase genes polymorphisms in genetic susceptibility to Philadelphia-negative myeloproliferative neoplasms in a Portuguese population. Pathology & Oncology Research. 2018; 1-9. DOI: 10.1007/s12253-018-0411-y

[112] Reuther GW. Myeloproliferative neoplasms: Molecular drivers and therapeutics. Progress in Molecular Biology and Translational Science. 2016;**144**:437-484

[113] Tefferi A, Pardanani A. JAK inhibitors in myeloproliferative neoplasms: Rationale, current data and perspective. Blood Reviews. 2011;**25**:229-237

[114] Ebid GT, Ghareeb M, Salaheldin O, Kamel MM. Prevalence of the frequency of JAK2 (V617F) mutation in different myeloproliferative disorders in Egyptian patients. International Journal of Clinical and Experimental Pathology. 2015;**8**:11555-11559

[115] Jatiani SS, Baker SJ, Silverman LR, Reddy EP. JAK/STAT pathways in cytokine signaling and myeloproliferative disorders: Approaches for targeted therapies. Genes & Cancer. 2010;**1**:979-993

[116] Anand S, Stedham F, Beer P, Gudgin E, Ortmann CA, Bench A, et al. Effects of the JAK2 mutation on the hematopoietic stem and progenitor compartment in human myeloproliferative neoplasms. Blood. 2011;**118**:177-181

[117] Steensma DP, McClure RF, Karp JE, Tefferi A, Lasho TL, Powell HL, et al. JAK2 V617F is a rare finding in de novo acute myeloid leukemia, but STAT3 activation is common and remains unexplained. Leukemia. 2006;**20**:971-978

[118] Green DR, Llambi F. Cell death signaling. Cold Spring Harb Perspect Biol. Dec 2015;7(12):a006080. DOI: 10.1101/cshperspect.a006080

[119] Chen E, Mullally A. How does JAK2V617F contribute to the pathogenesis of myeloproliferative neoplasms? Hematology. American Society of Hematology. Education Program. 2014;**2014**:268-276

[120] Vainchenker W, Kralovics R. Genetic basis and molecular pathophysiology of classical myeloproliferative neoplasms. Blood. 2017;**129**:667-679

[121] Michiels JJ. Clinical, pathological and molecular features of the chronic myeloproliferative disorders: MPD 2005 and beyond. Hematology. 2005;**10**(Suppl 1):215-223

[122] Yao H, Ma Y, Hong Z, Zhao L, Monaghan SA, Hu MC, et al. Activating JAK2 mutants reveal cytokine receptor coupling differences that impact outcomes in myeloproliferative neoplasm. Leukemia. 2017

[123] Vorechovsky I, Jones AV, Cross NC. Why do we see JAK2 exon 12 mutations in myeloproliferative neoplasms? Leukemia. 2013;**27**:1930-1932

[124] Godfrey AL, Chen E, Massie CE, Silber Y, Pagano F, Bellosillo B, et al. STAT1 activation in association with JAK2 exon 12 mutations. Haematologica. 2016;**101**:e15-e19

[125] Bolufer P, Barragan E, Collado M, Cervera J, López JA, Sanz MA. Influence of genetic polymorphisms on the risk of developing leukemia and on disease progression. Leukemia Research. 2006;**30**:1471-1491

[126] Beer PA, Delhommeau F, LeCouédic JP, Dawson MA, Chen E, Bareford D, et al. Two routes to leukemic transformation after a JAK2 mutation-positive myeloproliferative neoplasm. Blood. 2010;**115**:2891-2900

[127] Kilpivaara O, Levine RL. JAK2 and MPL mutations in myeloproliferative neoplasms: Discovery and science. Leukemia. 2008;**22**:1813-1817

[128] Björkholm M, Hultcrantz M, Derolf Å. Leukemic transformation in myeloproliferative neoplasms: Therapy-related or unrelated? Best Practice & Research. Clinical Haematology. 2014;**27**:141-153

[129] Rueff J, Rodrigues AS. Cancer drug resistance: A brief overview from a genetic viewpoint. Methods in Molecular Biology. 2016;**1395**:1-18

[130] Rice KL, Lin X, Wolniak K, Ebert BL, Berkofsky-Fessler W, Buzzai M, et al. Analysis of genomic aberrations and gene expression profiling identifies novel lesions and pathways in myeloproliferative neoplasms. Blood Cancer Journal. 2011;**1**:e40

[131] Campregher PV, Santos FP, Perini GF, Hamerschlak N. Molecular biology of Philadelphia-negative myeloproliferative neoplasms. Revista Brasileira de Hematologia e Hemoterapia. 2012;**34**:150-155

[132] Vannucchi AM, Antonioli E, Guglielmelli P, Rambaldi A, Barosi G, Marchioli R, et al. Clinical profile of homozygous JAK2 617V>F mutation in patients with polycythemia vera or essential thrombocythemia. Blood. 2007;**110**:840-846

[133] Pietra D, Li S, Brisci A, Passamonti F, Rumi E, Theocharides A, et al. Somatic mutations of JAK2 exon 12 in patients with JAK2 (V617F)-negative myeloproliferative disorders. Blood. 2008;**111**:1686-1689

[134] Passamonti F, Rumi E, Pietra D, Elena C, Boveri E, Arcaini L, et al. A prospective study of 338 patients with polycythemia vera: The impact of JAK2 (V617F) allele burden and leukocytosis on fibrotic or leukemic disease transformation and vascular complications. Leukemia. 2010;**24**:1574-1579

[135] Butcher CM, Hahn U, To LB, Gecz J, Wilkins EJ, Scott HS, et al. Two novel JAK2 exon 12 mutations in JAK2V617F-negative polycythaemia vera patients. Leukemia. 2008;**22**:870-873

[136] Rumi E, Pietra D, Ferretti V, Klampfl T, Harutyunyan AS, Milosevic JD, et al. JAK2 or CALR mutation status defines subtypes of essential thrombocythemia with substantially different clinical course and outcomes. Blood. 2014;**123**:1544-1551

[137] Scott LM, Beer PA, Bench AJ, Erber WN, Green AR. Prevalence of JAK2 V617F and exon 12 mutations in polycythaemia vera. British Journal of Haematology. 2007;**139**:511-512

[138] Scott LM. The JAK2 exon 12 mutations: A comprehensive review. American Journal of Hematology. 2011;**86**:668-676

[139] Park CH, Lee KO, Jang JH, Jung CW, Kim JW, Kim SH, et al. High frequency of JAK2 exon 12 mutations in Korean patients with polycythaemia vera: Novel mutations and clinical significance. Journal of Clinical Pathology. 2016;**69**:737-741

[140] Passamonti F, Elena C, Schnittger S, Skoda RC, Green AR, Girodon F, et al. Molecular and clinical features of the myeloproliferative neoplasm associated with JAK2 exon 12 mutations. Blood. 2011;**117**:2813-2816

[141] Pardanani A, Lasho TL, Finke C, Hanson CA, Tefferi A. Prevalence and clinicopathologic correlates of JAK2 exon 12 mutations in JAK2V617F-negative polycythemia vera. Leukemia. 2007;**21**:1960-1963

[142] Wu Z, Zhang X, Xu X, Chen Y, Hu T, Kang Z, et al. The mutation profile of JAK2 and CALR in Chinese Han patients with Philadelphia chromosome-negative myeloproliferative neoplasms. Journal of Hematology & Oncology. 2014;**7**:48

[143] Ishii T, Bruno E, Hoffman R, Xu M. Involvement of various hematopoietic-cell lineages by the JAK2V617F mutation in polycythemia vera. Blood. 2006;**108**:3128-3134

[144] Mousinho F, Santos PSE, Azevedo AP, Pereira JM, Lemos R, Matos S, et al. Concomitant myeloproliferative and lymphoproliferative neoplasms, distinct progenitors: A case report and review of the literature. Molecular and Clinical Oncology. 2018;**9**:347-349

[145] Mousinho F, Azevedo AP, Mendes T, Santos PSE, Cerqueira R, Matos S,et al. Concomitant

presence of JAK2V617F mutation and BCR-ABL translocation in two patients: A new entity or a variant of myeloproliferative neoplasms (Case report). Molecular Medicine Reports. 2018;**18**:1001-1006

[146] Vainchenker W, Constantinescu SN. JAK/STAT signaling in hematological malignancies. Oncogene. 2013;**32**:2601-2613

[147] Thomas SJ, Snowden JA, Zeidler MP, Danson SJ. The role of JAK/STAT signalling in the pathogenesis, prognosis and treatment of solid tumours. British Journal of Cancer. 2015;**113**:365-371

[148] Nielsen C, Birgens HS, Nordestgaard BG, Kjaer L, Bojesen SE. The JAK2 V617F somatic mutation, mortality and cancer risk in the general population. Haematologica. 2011;**96**:450-453

[149] Jaiswal S, Fontanillas P, Flannick J, Manning A, Grauman PV, Mar BG, et al. Age-related clonal hematopoiesis associated with adverse outcomes. The New England Journal of Medicine. 2014;**371**:2488-2498

[150] Nielsen C, Birgens HS, Nordestgaard BG, Bojesen SE. Diagnostic value of JAK2 V617F somatic mutation for myeloproliferative cancer in 49 488 individuals from the general population. British Journal of Haematology. 2013;**160**:70-79

[151] Nielsen C, Bojesen SE, Nordestgaard BG, Kofoed KF, Birgens HS. JAK2V617F somatic mutation in the general population: Myeloproliferative neoplasm development and progression rate. Haematologica. 2014;**99**:1448-1455

[152] Larsen TS, Pallisgaard N, Møller MB, Hasselbalch HC. The JAK2 V617F allele burden in essential thrombocythemia, polycythemia vera and primary myelofibrosis--impact on disease phenotype. European Journal of Haematology. 2007;**79**:508-515

[153] Vannucchi AM, Pieri L, Guglielmelli P. JAK2 allele burden in the myeloproliferative neoplasms: Effects on phenotype, prognosis and change with treatment. Therapeutic Advances in Hematology. 2011;**2**:21-32

[154] Duletić AN, Dekanić A, Hadzisejdić I, Kusen I, Matusan-Ilijas K, Grohovac D, et al. JAK2-v617F mutation is associated with clinical and laboratory features of myeloproliferative neoplasms. Collegium Antropologicum. 2012;**36**:859-865

[155] Ha JS, Kim YK, Jung SI, Jung HR, Chung IS. Correlations between Janus kinase 2 V617F allele burdens and clinicohematologic parameters in myeloproliferative neoplasms. Annals of Laboratory Medicine. 2012;**32**:385-391

[156] Pardanani A, Lasho T, McClure R, Lacy M, Tefferi A. Discordant distribution of JAK2V617F mutation in siblings with familial myeloproliferative disorders. Blood. 2006;**107**:4572-4573

[157] Jones AV, Kreil S, Zoi K, Waghorn K, Curtis C, Zhang L, et al. Widespread occurrence of the JAK2 V617F mutation in chronic myeloproliferative disorders. Blood. 2005;**106**:2162-2168

[158] Lundberg P, Takizawa H, Kubovcakova L, Guo G, Hao-Shen H, Dirnhofer S, et al. Myeloproliferative neoplasms can be initiated from a single hematopoietic stem cell expressing JAK2-V617F. The Journal of Experimental Medicine. 2014;**211**:2213-2230

[159] Bastos HN, Antão MR, Silva SN, Azevedo AP, Manita I, Teixeira V, et al. Association of polymorphisms in genes of the homologous recombination DNA repair pathway and thyroid cancer risk. Thyroid. 2009;**19**:1067-1075

[160] Conde J, Silva SN, Azevedo AP, Teixeira V, Pina JE, Rueff J, et al. Association of common variants in mismatch repair genes and breast cancer susceptibility: A multigene study. BMC Cancer. 2009;**9**:344

[161] Barbui T, Vannucchi AM, Buxhofer-Ausch V, De Stefano V, Betti S, Rambaldi A, et al. Practice-relevant revision of IPSET-thrombosis based on 1019 patients with WHO-defined essential thrombocythemia. Blood Cancer Journal. 2015;**5**:e369

[162] Guglielmelli P, Lasho TL, Rotunno G, Score J, Mannarelli C, Pancrazzi A, et al. The number of prognostically detrimental mutations and prognosis in primary myelofibrosis: An international study of 797 patients. Leukemia. 2014;**28**:1804-1810

[163] Theocharides A, Boissinot M, Girodon F, Garand R, Teo SS, Lippert E, et al. Leukemic blasts in transformed JAK2-V617F-positive myeloproliferative disorders are frequently negative for the JAK2-V617F mutation. Blood. 2007;**110**:375-379

[164] Barbui T, Finazzi G, Falanga A. Myeloproliferative neoplasms and thrombosis. Blood. 2013;**122**:2176-2184

[165] Carobbio A, Finazzi G, Guerini V, Spinelli O, Delaini F, Marchioli R, et al. Leukocytosis is a risk factor for thrombosis in essential thrombocythemia: Interaction with treatment, standard risk factors, and JAK2 mutation status. Blood. 2007;**109**:2310-2313

[166] Tefferi A, Vannucchi AM. Genetic risk assessment in myeloproliferative neoplasms. Mayo Clinic Proceedings. 2017;**92**:1283-1290

[167] Hernández-Boluda JC, Pereira A, Cervantes F, Alvarez-Larrán A, Collado M, Such E, et al. A polymorphism in the XPD gene predisposes to leukemic transformation and new nonmyeloid malignancies in essential thrombocythemia and polycythemia vera. Blood. 2012;**119**:5221-5228

[168] Pardanani A, Fridley BL, Lasho TL, Gilliland DG, Tefferi A. Host genetic variation contributes to phenotypic diversity in myeloproliferative disorders. Blood. 2008;**111**:2785-2789

[169] Lasho TL, Tefferi A, Hood JD, Verstovsek S, Gilliland DG, Pardanani A. TG101348, a JAK2-selective antagonist, inhibits primary hematopoietic cells derived from myeloproliferative disorder patients with JAK2V617F, MPLW515K or JAK2 exon 12 mutations as well as mutation negative patients. Leukemia. 2008;**22**:1790-1792

[170] Harrison C, Kiladjian JJ, Al-Ali HK, Gisslinger H, Waltzman R, Stalbovskaya V, et al. JAK inhibition with ruxolitinib versus best available therapy for myelofibrosis. The New England Journal of Medicine. 2012;**366**:787-798

[171] Verstovsek S, Mesa RA, Gotlib J, Levy RS, Gupta V, DiPersio JF, et al. A double-blind, placebo-controlled trial of ruxolitinib for myelofibrosis. The New England Journal of Medicine. 2012;**366**:799-807

[172] Hobbs GS, Rozelle S, Mullally A. The development and use of Janus kinase 2 inhibitors for the treatment of myeloproliferative neoplasms. Hematology/Oncology Clinics of North America. 2017;**31**:613-626

[173] Vannucchi AM, Harrison CN. Emerging treatments for classical myeloproliferative neoplasms. Blood. 2017;**129**:693-703

[174] Stahl M, Zeidan AM. Management of myelofibrosis: JAK inhibition and beyond. Expert Review of Hematology. 2017;**10**:459-477

Chapter 3

JAK, an Oncokinase in Hematological Cancer

Carlota Recio, Haidée Aranda-Tavío,
Miguel Guerra-Rodríguez,
Mercedes de Mirecki-Garrido, Patricia Martín-Rodríguez,
Borja Guerra and Leandro Fernández-Pérez

Abstract

Janus kinases (JAKs) play an essential role in the regulation of cytokine signaling. They control cell survival, proliferation, differentiation, immune response, and hematopoiesis. Deregulation of JAK signaling has been associated to the pathogenesis of numerous immune-inflammatory diseases, hematological malignancies, and solid tumors. Thus, JAK proteins have emerged as attractive therapeutic targets in the last decade. The discovery of the gain-of-function JAK2 mutation (JAK2 V617F) as the main cause of polycythemia vera—a chronic myeloproliferative syndrome—led to the development of the JAK inhibitor ruxolitinib. This key finding opened the door to the search for new therapeutic agents able to suppress the constitutive activation of JAK signaling in hematological cancers and other tumors. However, given the conserved nature of the kinase domain among JAK family members, and the interrelated roles of JAK kinases in many physiological processes, including hematopoiesis and immunity, the broad usage of JAK inhibitors in hematology is challenged by their narrow therapeutic window. Novel therapies are, therefore, needed. This chapter focuses on the understanding of the complex signaling of JAK proteins in cancerous cells, the various JAK aberrations implicated in myeloproliferative neoplasms, leukemia, and lymphoma, and the clinically available JAK inhibitors in cancer therapy.

Keywords: blood cancer, hematological tumor, JAK, STAT, mutation, JAK2 V617F

1. Introduction

The Janus kinase (JAK) signal transducer and activators of transcription (STAT) intracellular pathway connects the signaling from extracellular cytokines, hormones, and growth factors, with the nuclear transcriptional machinery [1]. It is expressed in animals from flies to humans, being highly evolutionarily conserved [2]. The cascade consists of the tyrosine kinase JAK, the transcription factor STAT, and different regulatory proteins. In mammals, four JAKs and seven STATs have been identified [3]. JAK/STAT signaling controls numerous essential cellular responses, including cell proliferation, differentiation, migration, immune response, apoptosis, and cell survival, according to the signal, cell context, and tissue [4, 5]. These cellular events are crucial to a wide range of biological functions like hematopoiesis, immune development, inflammatory response, adipogenesis, and angiogenesis, among others [6]. Under normal physiological conditions, JAK/STAT pathway signaling is strictly regulated. However, in different pathological conditions such as cancer, atherosclerosis, rheumatoid arthritis, or diabetes, an "aberrant" regulation of JAK/STAT signaling has been described [6]. Mutations on JAK proteins have been reported in certain cancers, highlighting hematological cancers (HCs). Generally, these are JAK gain-of-function mutations that promote constitutive STAT activation, which triggers tumorigenesis, high-grade inflammation, or hypergrowing, among other pathological consequences [7]. As consequence, JAK inhibitors are gaining prominence in clinical use, mainly in the treatment of HCs driven by JAK mutations, or in those tumors in which JAK/STAT pathway is determinant for the pathogenesis [8, 9]. Interestingly, not only in HCs therapy, but also in the treatment of advanced solid tumors such as pancreatic cancer and triple-negative breast cancer, and certain autoimmune and inflammatory diseases such as rheumatoid arthritis, JAK inhibitors are under clinical trial [10, 11].

2. The JAK/STAT pathway

2.1 JAKs

JAK proteins are nonreceptor tyrosine kinases that are essential for the activation of signaling mediated by receptors for cytokines, hormones, or several growth factors. The family includes four 120–130 kDa proteins, named JAK1, JAK2, JAK3, and TYK2, with seven defined regions of homology, called JAK homology (JH) domains (JH1–JH7) [5] (**Figure 1**). The C-terminal region includes the kinase (JH1) and the pseudokinase (JH2) domains. JH1 domain contains tyrosine residues in the activation loop, essential for JAK activation. The pseudokinase domain JH2 is structurally analogous to JH1 and participates on its activity regulation but lacks characteristic residues of tyrosine kinases, which makes it catalytically inactive [12]. Next, the SH2-related domain is constituted by JH3 and part of JH4; this region mediates JAK docking to phosphorylated tyrosine residues [13]. The other half of JH4 to JH7 domains compose the N-terminal region, called FERM (four-point-one, ezrin, radixin, and moesin), which are involved in the association between JAK and cytokine receptors [12].

2.2 STATs

The STAT family consists of seven members, named STAT1 to STAT4, STAT5A, STAT5B, and STAT6, of 80–100 kDa, which share highly conserved homology

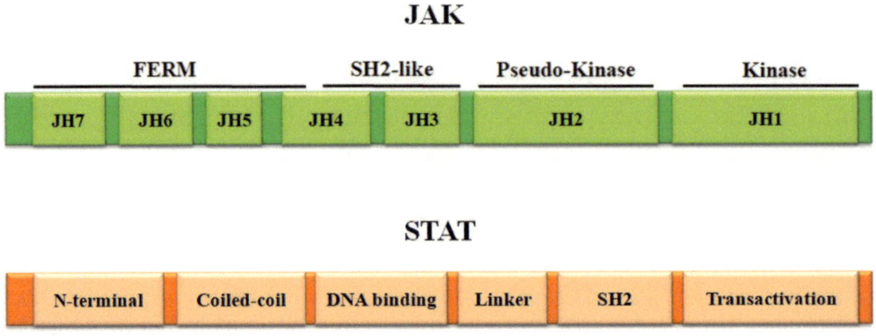

Figure 1.
JAKs and STATs structural domains.

regions. These include (a) an N-terminal domain, (b) a spiral domain, (c) a DNA-binding domain, (d) a SH2 domain, and (e) a transactivation domain at the C-terminal end [7] (**Figure 1**). The N-terminal region is the less conserved one among the STATs, and it is implicated in some STAT dimer-dimer and other protein interactions. The spiral coiled-coil domain is responsible for many other protein-protein interactions [6]. The STAT binding to DNA is mediated by the DNA-binding domain, which defines that STAT dimers recognize an 8- to 10-base pair inverted repeat DNA element with a consensus sequence of 5′-TTCN2–4GAA-3′. Differential binding affinity of an activated STAT dimer for a single target DNA sequence is determined by the number of nucleotides between TTC and GAA [14]. The SH2 domain is responsible to target STATs to specific tyrosine-phosphorylated peptide sequences within their binding molecules, thus controlling a broad range of intracellular signaling functions [7]. The transactivation domain holds two aminoacidic residues (tyrosine and serine) essential for STAT activity; so that JAK-promoted tyrosine phosphorylation leads to STAT dimerization, whereas STAT serine phosphorylation mediated by mitogen-activated protein kinases (MAPKs) enhances its transcriptional activity [7, 15]. All these domains are essential for STAT biological functions in response to extracellular stimuli such as cytokines or growth factors.

2.3 Pathway signaling

External stimuli (i.e., cytokines, growth factors) bind their receptors in the cellular membrane activating receptor-associated JAK autophosphorylation and subsequent activation. This event triggers a conformational change in JAK structure, which gets it ready for binding substrate and exerting its kinase activity. JAK binding sites are then exposed to the cytoplasm, where STAT monomers are found themselves in latency. STATs are recruited to the recognition areas at JAK-binding sites being phosphorylated by JAKs, which triggers their dimerization in homodimers (STAT1, STAT3, STAT4, STAT5A, and STAT5B) or heterodimers (STAT1-STAT2 and STAT1-STAT3). Consequently, active STAT dimers translocate into the nucleus where they bind to DNA, activating or repressing the transcription of their target genes [3, 6] (**Figure 2**). According to the cellular context, the external stimuli implicated, and the receptors engaged, different JAKs and STATs can be activated [16, 17] (**Table 1**).

Interestingly, through a noncanonical signaling, other tyrosine kinases different from JAKs can activate STAT factors, including membrane-bound growth factor receptor tyrosine kinases (e.g., epidermal growth factor receptor—EGFR, platelet derived growth factor receptor—PDGFR) and nonreceptor tyrosine kinases (e.g., the proto-oncogene tyrosine kinases Src and Bcr-Abl) [2, 18]. Furthermore, STAT has been shown to be able to form dimers and exert biological activity in absence of canonical JAK tyrosine phosphorylation [19]. In fact, activated JAK2 has been reported that it can enter the nucleus where it mediates epigenetic modifications of histones [20]. Furthermore, a fraction of inactive STAT5 has been found to be localized in the nucleus (instead of in the cytoplasm as the canonical signaling describes), where it is not susceptible of being phosphorylated by tyrosine kinases, mediating chromatin stabilization [21, 22].

2.4 Regulation of JAK/STAT pathway

Owing to the implication of JAK/STAT pathway in many relevant biological processes, its endogenous regulation is tight and precise. Besides, since deregulated JAKs and STATs have been associated with several pathological disorders, most of JAK/STAT modulators have been largely assessed as interesting therapeutic approaches. One of the conventional JAK/STAT modulators is protein tyrosine

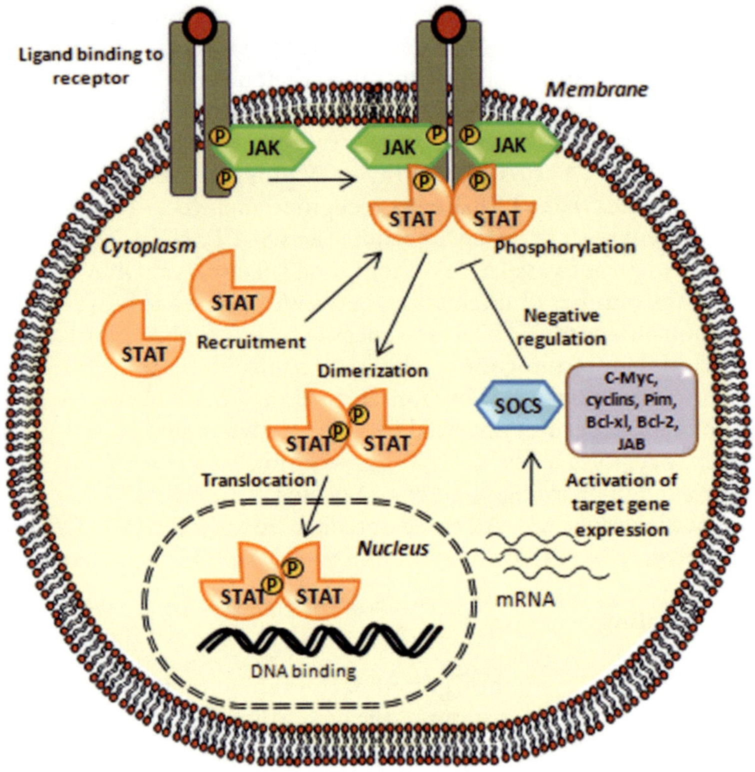

Figure 2.
JAK/STAT signaling pathway.

Cytokine/growth factor	Activated JAK	Activated STAT	Therapeutic area
IFN (α,β,γ)	JAK1, JAK2, TYK2	STAT1, STAT2	Immune regulation, cancer
IL-10	JAK1, TYK2	STAT1, STAT3	Immune regulation
IL-2, IL-7, IL-9, IL-15	JAK1, JAK3	STAT5, STAT3	Immune regulation, asthma
IL-4, IL-13	JAK1, JAK2, JAK3	STAT6	Allergy, asthma
IL-3, IL-5, GM-CSF	JAK2	STAT5	Myeloid reconstitution, asthma
IL-12, G-CSF, EPO, TPO, PRL, GH	JAK2, JAK1, TYK2	STAT5, STAT3, STAT4, STAT1	Immune regulation, myeloid reconstitution, anemia, platelet production, growth, aging
CSF-1/M-CSF, EGF, PDGF, insulin	JAK1	STAT1, STAT3, STAT5	Cancer, diabetes
IL-6, IL-11, leptin, CT-1	JAK2, JAK1, TYK2	STAT1, STAT3, STAT5	Inflammation, platelet production, obesity, cardiovascular disease

Table 1.
Differential activation of JAK/STAT pathway upon ligand binding.

phosphatases (PTPs), which negatively regulate the signaling of the pathway by dephosphorylating the JAK-associated receptor and/or JAK itself. Furthermore, the protein inhibitors of activated STATs (PIAS) constitute another classical group of JAK/STAT negative regulators. This family of proteins can inhibit STAT signaling and function by directly preventing STAT from binding DNA or indirectly inhibiting STAT dimerization [23, 24]. But doubtlessly, the most broadly studied group of negative modulators of JAK/STAT signaling is the family of Suppressor of Cytokine Signaling (SOCS) proteins [25]. The family comprises eight members (SOCS1–7 and CIS) of 20–30 kDa, which show different structural domains including a N-terminal domain of variable length, little conserved; a central Src homology region that contains an extended SH2 sequence that leads to SOCS binding to tyrosine-phosphorylated residues either on the associated receptor or at JAK protein; and a highly conserved C-terminal domain, called SOCS box [25, 26]. Furthermore, SOCS1 and SOCS3 share a small kinase inhibitory region (KIR) located at their N-terminal region, which is implicated in the inhibition of JAK-catalytic activity. SOCS proteins exert a negative feedback loop mechanism, so that activated STATs induce the expression of SOCS, which then control STAT transduction signaling (**Figure 2**). The mechanisms by which SOCS proteins suppress JAK/STAT signaling include (1) binding to JAK catalytic site and subsequent inhibition of its kinase activity; (2) competition with STAT for the binding sites on the associated receptor; and (3) proteasomal degradation [23].

3. JAK in hematopoiesis

Hematopoiesis is a multistep process by which blood cells, which have a limited life span, are continuously renewed. It is initiated in the bone marrow with the proliferation and differentiation of pluripotent hematopoietic stem cells, which undergo asymmetric divisions and differentiate into lineage-committed progenitors that eventually give rise to specialized blood cells [9]. Deregulation in hematopoiesis leads to the accumulation of intermediate progenitors or mature cells in the bone marrow, blood, or lymphoid tissues driving hematological malignancies [9]. Hematopoietic cytokines including erythropoietin (EPO), thrombopoietin (TPO), granulocyte colony-stimulating factor (GM-CSF), among others, tightly regulate hematopoiesis. They maintain regular levels of blood cells or induce their production according to physiological needs. These cytokines bind to their cognate receptors at the cell membrane, which generally (except some tyrosine kinases such as c-KIT, FLT-3, or GM-CSF receptor) lack intrinsic enzymatic activity at their intracellular part. Nevertheless, these receptor chains are constitutively associated with a JAK kinase, which mediates cytokine-induced signaling [9]. During myelopoiesis, JAK2 has been found to respond upon EPO, TPO, G-CSF, GM-CSF, IL-3, and IL-5 binding, mediating myeloid cell proliferation and differentiation [9], whereas in lymphopoiesis are mainly JAK1 and JAK3, which cooperate by binding to specific cytokine receptors (IL-2R, IL-4R, IL-7R and IL-15R). It has been suggested that JAK1 functions as the primary signaling effector since JAK3 is a JAK1 scaffold [9]. Gene disruption studies have confirmed the essential role of JAK proteins in hematopoiesis. JAK1-deficient mice showed perinatal lethality and defective lymphoid development [27]. Lack of JAK2 expression resulted in an embryonic lethality due to a block in erythropoiesis but with intact lymphoid development [27]. JAK3 deficiency revealed severe combined immunodeficiency with low functional T and B cell numbers and aberrant myelopoiesis [27].

4. Aberrant JAK signaling and hematological cancer development

The multifactorial process of tumorigenesis is characterized by cellular fail in sensing and repairing DNA damage, loss of regulation of cell cycle progression and apoptosis, and expression of aberrant patterns of growth signaling and angiogenesis [28, 29]. Numerous studies have provided strong evidence for the key role that JAK kinases play in hematologic cancer genesis and progression. This is not surprising considering the close relation between JAKs and cytokine and growth factor signaling, hematopoiesis, proliferation, apoptosis, and immune response, processes that, when deregulated, contribute to tumor development [29, 30]. Either gain-of-function mutations in JAKs, cognate JAK tyrosine kinases, or JAK associate receptors, the generation of fusion proteins, or the loss of negative feedback regulation of JAK signaling can contribute to constitutive and aberrant STAT signaling and therefore to oncogenesis [18]. The first evidence of the strong implication of JAK kinases in HCs was the identification of oncogenic fusion proteins involving JAK kinase domain (e.g., TEL/ETV6-JAK2) [31]. Subsequently, other JAK2 fusion proteins and JAK2 gene amplifications have been identified. However, although they were more recently discovered, JAK point somatic mutations are the most common JAK deregulations found in hematological tumors, being the mutation JAK2 V617F found in more than half of all classical myeloproliferative disorders (MPDs) [32]. Besides, other JAK mutations are associated to hematological malignancies, such as JAK1 mutations, found in 10–20% of T-ALL, and other JAK2 mutations associated to ~20% of Down syndrome (DS)-associated B-ALL [32] (**Table 2**). Interestingly, the discovery of all these mutations has highlighted JAK proteins as potent drug targets and biomarkers for HCs.

4.1 JAK2 mutations

4.1.1 JAK2V617F mutation in myeloproliferative disorders

Myeloproliferative disorders (MPDs) are a group of chronic clonal malignancies arising from the expansion of mature hematopoietic progenitor cells [33]. The World Health Organization (WHO) distinguishes two MPDs subtypes: (a) chronic myelogenous leukemia (CML) involving the Philadelphia (Ph) chromosome, frequently associated to BCR-ABL fusion oncoprotein and (b) a set of Ph-negative MPDs syndromes mainly referred to polycythemia vera (PV), essential thrombocythemia (ET), and idiopathic myelofibrosis (IMF) [34]. Two key features of this second group are the ability of cytokine-independent blood colony formation [33, 35] and hypersensitivity to numerous cytokines [36, 37]. However, each subtype is characterized by the clonal production of different hematologic lineages. PV and ET present, for example, an increased production of platelets and red cells. Accumulating evidences over the last decade establish that Ph-negative MPDs frequently carry a JAK2 single point somatic mutation at chromosome 9p24, exon 14

JAK	Mutation	Associated disease
JAK2	V617F	MPDs
	K539L	PV
	T875N	Acute megakaryoblastic myeloid leukemia
	Deletion of IREED	ALL
JAK1	A634D	T-ALL
	T478S, V623A	AML
JAK3	A572V, V722I, P132T	Acute megakaryoblastic myeloid leukemia

Table 2.
Mutation in human JAKs and disease association.

(JAK2V617F—Val617Phe) [38, 39]. This genetic abnormality has stem cell nature, affecting all cells of the myeloid lineages [36, 40], whereas clonal involvement of the lymphoid lineage is controversial, and its effects are less understood. Larsen and colleagues detected the JAK2V617F mutation in both B lymphocytes and T lymphocytes in a subgroup of patients with Ph-negative MPDs. Their results suggested an early stem cell origin with both lymphoid and myeloid differentiation possibilities [41]. JAK2V617F mutation is present in 50–60% of patients with ET and IMF and in most of cases of PV [35, 36, 40]. Some reports have also related JAK2V617F mutation to other myeloid malignancies like chronic myelomonocytic leukemia (CMML), myelodysplasia (MD), and, in rare cases, acute myelogenous leukemia (AML) [42]. Additionally, in other less frequent leukemias like mediastinal B cell lymphoma and Hodgkin lymphoma, both with amplification of the JAK2V617F mutation, researchers were conscious about an epigenetic role of aberrant JAK2 kinase, leading to histone H3 phosphorylation, thereby promoting gene expression [43]. The origin of JAK2V617F mutation is localized within the pseudokinase domain, JH2 of JAK2 gene [36]. JAK2 activation requires Y1007 phosphorylation [33] and its activation is crucial for cytokine-mediated signaling from the EPO receptor and other type I cytokine receptors [44]. In this sense, JAK2V617F somatic mutation is phosphorylated at Y1007, conferring constitutive activation of JAK2 tyrosine kinase by decreasing the autoinhibitory effect of JH2, thereby recapitulating cytokine receptor downstream signaling pathways, among these STAT5 and ERK (extracellular signal-regulated kinase) [33, 35, 45] (**Figure 3**). The discovery could be performed by tyrosine kinase gene sequencing in MPD patients [35, 36] and by assessing the role of JAK2V617F mutation in different in vitro studies. Cellular transformation of cytokine-dependent cell lines like Ba/F3, Ba/F3-EpoR, and FDCP-EpoR with JAK2 mutant variant led to cytokine-independent signaling triggered by JAK2 constitutive phosphorylation and induced erythrocytosis; whereas concomitant wild-type JAK2 overexpression restored or alternatively decreased the effects of the mutation in vitro [35, 40]. Lower levels of JAK2V617F required coexpression of dimeric type 1 cytokine receptor as a scaffold for the independence of hormone signaling status in Ba/F3 cells [46]. Retroviral transplant mouse models have evidenced that JAK2V617F presence is enough for reproducing PV and IMF diseases in vivo [33, 35, 46]. However, its related effects on ET remained insufficiently understood [45], exposing no sufficient JAK2V617F influence on platelet number [44, 47].

Three hypotheses have been suggested for explaining the causes of phenotype variability exhibited by JAK2V617F: gene dosage background, unidentified mutations, and receptor interaction with JAK2 during myeloid and erythroid differentiation [35, 42]. In the first case, mice genotyping of the JAK2V617F gene showed increased expression of this protein in homozygote samples, leading to PV or IMF like diseases. Homozygous form of this single-point mutation is found in at least 30% of PV patients, probably due to mitotic recombination [36, 40]. On the other

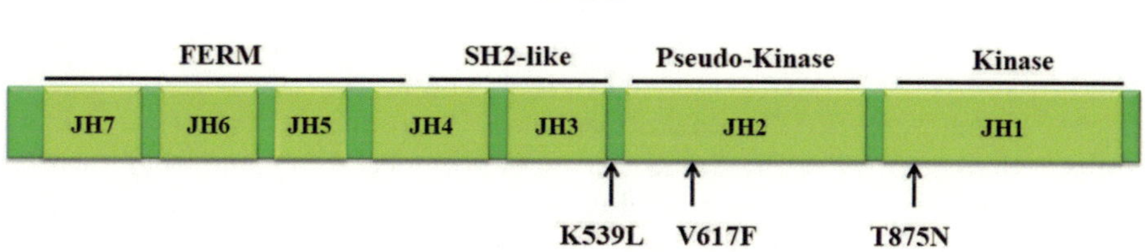

Figure 3.
JAK2 point mutations.

hand, heterozygous mice might drive the ET phenotype. In fact, data point out ET as the most heterogeneous MPD. The second hypothesis suggests that the precedence or upcoming sequence of nonidentified mutations following JAK2V617F may drive the acquisition of one or another phenotype [40, 42], thus showing genetic heterogeneity [35]. Finally, Funakoshi and colleagues proposed that cellular context-specific receptor's interaction with JAK2V617F expression levels would determine the activated phenotype [48]. From another perspective, JAK2V617F mutation in Ph-negative MPDs leads to constitutive phosphorylation of JAK2 in the absence of EPO [36]. This event is closely linked to downstream STAT3/5 proteins phosphorylation. PV patients exhibit high STAT5 and STAT3 phosphorylation; ET patients exhibit high STAT3 but low STAT5 phosphorylation; and myelofibrosis patients exhibit both low STAT5 and STAT3 phosphorylation. Different STAT3/5 phosphorylation patterns allow the discrimination among Ph-negative MPDs [49]. As we can see, constitutive activation of JAK2–STAT5 or JAK2–STAT3 signaling is a major driver of PV, ET, and IMF [36, 49]. In short, JAK/STAT signaling pathway is demonstrated to be essential for hematologic stem cells differentiation. Focusing on JAK2 as a therapeutically valid target remains an attractive option for MPDs treatment.

4.1.2 JAK2K539L mutation (exon 12 mutations) in polycythemia vera

The JAK2V617F mutation discovery was followed by other different JAK2 gene gain-of-function mutations identification [33, 38, 50–52]. As we have already described above, most PV patients express JAK2V617F [36, 40, 52]. Nevertheless, less frequently (3–5%) PV cases harbor several exon 12 JAK2 mutations present in the linking region of JH2 and JH3 domains, encompassing a highly conserved amino acid region F537–E543 in the absence of V617F mutation. This leads to a distinct clinical syndrome with isolated erythrocytosis [43, 53]. Three of the cluster of different JAK2 exon 12 mutations [43, 51, 52] included a substitution of leucine for lysine at position 539 (539L) of JAK2 in JAK2V617F-negative PV patients or idiopathic erythrocytosis: F537-K539delinsL, H538QK539L, and K539L. They are reported to be acquired, thus explaining why they appeared in peripheral-blood granulocytes but are absent in T lymphocytes [43, 51]. Functionally, K539L exon 12 mutations modify JH2 domain, resulting in aberrant growth factor responses in Ba/F3 cells *in vitro*. This cell line was able to proliferate without the addition of IL-3 and demonstrated to have an increased phosphorylation of JAK2, ERK1/2, and STAT5, in comparison to murine cells transduced by wild-type JAK2 or V617F JAK2 [39, 51, 54]. Furthermore, these mutations discharged a myeloproliferative phenotype in a murine model, resulting in higher levels of phosphorylated JAK2 compared to those with the V617F mutation. The described consequences as well as kinetics exhibited by K539L mutations were not distinguishable from those observed for cells with the V617F mutation [51]. From a genetic point of view, unlike JAK2V617F-positive PV patients, JAK2 exon 12-mutated PV patients are often heterozygous. However, they share a similar clinical outcome [39, 51].

4.1.3 JAK2T875N mutation in acute megakaryoblastic myeloid leukemia

Acute megakaryoblastic myeloid leukemia (AMKL) is a rare subtype of acute myeloid leukemia (AML) that presents different genetic characteristics and morphological phenotypes. AMKL appears frequently in childhood but is also common in adults in their 50s or 60s [55]. Some cases are developed after chemotherapy or are the result of leukemic transformation of chronic myeloproliferative neoplasms [56]. Diverse cytogenic abnormalities are associated to AMKL that differs between children and adults. The most commonly seen aberrations in adulthood are inv(3)(q21;q26), deletions of chromosomes 5 and 7, and t(9;22)(q34;q11) [55]. Children that develop this disease are subdivided in two groups. The first one presents constitutional trisomy 21 (Down syndrome) associated to a somatic mutation in *GATA-1* [57]. The second is represented by 1(1:22)(p13:q13) translocation that encodes a fusion protein OTT-MAL (RBM15-MKL1) [58]. Despite all these genetic factors, the fact that DS children spontaneously experiment disease remission, in most cases [57] together with the fact that models of GATA1 mutation fail in reproduce AMKL leukemogenesis [59], suggests that there should be several mechanisms contributing to AMKL promotion.

Merchel et al. were interested in the STAT5 hyperactivation observed in AML, which, in most cases, is the result of activating mutations in tyrosine kinases. In 2006, they identified a novel mutation in JAK2 studying AMKL cell lines such as CHRF-288-11, M07e, or UT7. DNA sequencing of all JAK family members in CHRF-288-11 detected a single homozygous JAK2C2624A allele. This mutation leads to a substitution of a threonine for an asparagine at position 875 of the JAK2 JH1 kinase domain (**Figure 3**). Based on the crystal structure of JAK2, T875 lies within the loop between strands β2 and β3, which could alter JH1-JH2 interface [56]. However, studying full-length JAK2 crystal structure is necessary to better comprehend the mechanism of constitutive activation of JAK2 mutants [60]. The other cell lines studied, M07e and UT7 (6-month-old and 64-year-old AMKL patients, respectively), did not express hyperactivated STAT5, which is consistent with the heterogeneity of this disorder [56]. Although the frequency of this mutation in patients remains unknown, everything points to an important role of JAK2T875N in AMKL. Indeed, this mutation constitutively activates JAK2 kinase and its downstream effectors in naturally carrying JAK2T875N mutation cells *in vitro* [56] and Ba/F3 cells transduced with EpoR or TpoR. Interestingly, this mutation conferred Ba/F3 cells the capacity of IL-3 independent growth [56, 60]. Moreover, comparative studies of Ba/F3 stably expressing JAK2 wild type or JAK2V617F, JAK2K539L, JAK2T875N mutations showed that the highest kinase activity is associated with JAK2T875N mutation followed by JAK2V617F [60]. Also, JAK2T875N expression was accompanied by significantly increased activation of pathways induced by cytokines and growth factors compared with the other mutations [60]. However, these differences were not detected in HEK293 cells expressing the same JAK2 mutants, which could be result of differences in the transduced cell type [61]. Surprisingly, the higher activation of JAK2-associated JAK2T875N mutant was not linked with the capacity of transforming erythroid progenitors in bone marrow, which showed to be the lowest among the other JAK2 mutations [60]. Moreover, expression of JAK2T875N in a murine bone marrow transplant model was able to reproduce myeloproliferative disease with some AMKL characteristics, except thrombocytosis, insinuating that other genetic events could be involved in the promotion of the disease [56].

4.1.4 JAK2 deletion of IREED (682–686) in acute lymphoblastic leukemia

Children with Down syndrome have an increased risk of developing ALL apart from AMKL, but unlike AMKL favorable outcomes, Down syndrome-ALL undergo higher toxicity of chemotherapy, leading to increased morbidity and mortality compared with non-Down syndrome ALL patients [62]. Activating JAK2 mutations are detected in approximately 20% of Down syndrome-ALL patients [63]. For this reason, Malinge et al. analyzed 90 cases of acute leukemia of myeloid or B-cell origin to screen activating gene mutations based on high level gene expression. This technique allowed them to discover a novel JAK2 mutation in a Down syndrome 4-year-old patient with B-cell precursor acute lymphoblastic leukemia (BCP-ALL). This JAK2 mutation encodes a protein that lacks five amino acids (682–686), JAK2ΔIREED. They confirmed constitutive activation of JAK-STAT, ERK, and AKT signaling pathways in Ba/F3 cells artificially harboring JAK2ΔIREED and

JAK2V216F mutations. As observed for other JAK2 mutations, EpoR expression was necessary for JAK2ΔIREED to transform Ba/F3 cells to growth factor independency. Remarkably, these cells were sensitive to the JAK inhibitor I. In addition, a bone marrow transplant in mice revealed that this mutation promoted MPD in the model, with increased platelet, granulocytic, and red blood cell counts. Intriguingly, EpoR, myeloproliferative leukemia (MPL), and G-CSF receptor are not transcribed in the patient's cells. Hence, which cytokine receptor chain expressed in the leukemic cells is likely to associate with the mutated JAK2 is still unclear [64]. Another important source of information was the study performed by Bercovich et al. that analyzed JAK2 DNA mutations on diagnostic bone marrow samples of 88 Down syndrome-ALL patients and 216 patients with sporadic ALL. They identified acquired somatic mutations of JAK2 in 18% of Down syndrome-ALL patients. Five different alleles were detected, affecting the same evolutionary conserved arginine residue (R683), which is predicted to be located at the pseudokinase to Src homology 2 domain interface. These mutations presented associated genotype-phenotype specificity. Jak2 mutant expression in Ba/F3 EpoR and TpoR cells conferred cytokine independent growth and constitutive activation of JAK2 and STAT5. They also described pro-B cells transduced with the R683S JAK2 as sensitive to pharmacological inhibition of JAK/STAT pathway [63]. Supporting these findings, another group recently performed a genetic study of 83 BCP-ALL cell lines, detecting activating JAK2 mutations in YCUB-5 cell line (JAK2 R683I) and KOPN49 cell line (JAK2 R683G) accompanied by RAS mutations, which point out the involvement of RAS pathway apart from JAK/STAT in the progression of the disease [65]. Furthermore, some reports showed that JAK2 and P2RY8-CRLF2 (cytokine receptor-like factor 2) mutations are rare in Japanese non-Down syndrome ALL and Down syndrome-ALL patients, while in Western countries, CRLF2 is overexpressed in approximately 50–60% of Down syndrome-ALL patients. JAK2 mutations and CRLF2 seem to act in conjunction in leukemogenesis. For this reason, it is being suggested that these genetic aberrations are related to ethnicity [63].

4.2 JAK3 mutations

As we mentioned above, JAK3 is involved in lymphocyte development and function, and to carry out its functions, JAK3 interacts with the common gamma chain of some interleukin receptors, including interleukin (IL)–2, IL-4, IL-7, IL-9, IL-15, and IL-21 [5, 66]. Recently, JAK3-activating mutations have been reported in different lymphoproliferative disorders [66–68]. Mutations within the FERM domain, essential for binding of JAK to its receptor, and defects in gamma chain of receptors involved in JAK3 signaling pathway are associated with severe combined immunodeficiency (SCID) [5] and X-linked SCID (XSCID) [69], respectively. There are several activating mutations of JAK3, which have been validated in Ba/F3 cells, including P132T, L156P, R172Q, E183G, Q501H, M511I, A572V, A573V, R657Q, and V722I [67]. Among these transforming mutations, some of them have been more extensively studied because of their frequency and pathological consequences.

4.2.1 JAK3A572V, V722I, P132T mutations in acute megakaryoblastic leukemia

In acute megakaryoblastic leukemia (AMKL), AMKL cells present constitutive STAT5 phosphorylation, which indicates an upstream tyrosine kinase activation. The identified candidate responsible of STAT5 activation was JAK3, which carried an A572V mutation in the pseudokinase JH2 [70] that negatively regulates the JH1 kinase activity. Analysis of the entire coding sequence of JAK3 in AMKL patients allowed for the identification of two additional JAK3 mutations: V722I substitution in the JH2 pseudokinase domain and P132T change in the JH6 domain of the receptor-binding region. These mutations resulted in constitutive activation of JAK3 and phosphorylation of STAT5 and made Ba/F3 hematopoietic cell line cytokine grow independently [66, 70, 71]. However, JAK3 A572V summarized some, but not all, of the phenotypic characteristics of AMKL in a murine bone marrow transplant model, suggesting that other mutations may cooperate in complete AMKL transformation [70].

4.2.2 JAK3A572V and A573V mutations in natural killer/T cell lymphoma

Natural killer/T cell lymphoma (NKTCL) is a localized (areas of Asian and South America) aggressive subtype of non-Hodgkin lymphoma, with molecular characteristics and pathogenesis quite unknown. JAK3A572V and JAK3A573V mutations, located at exon 12 in the JH2 domain, have been described associated to this disease [67, 72]. NK cells need interleukin (IL)-2 to proliferate and be activated and this cytokine mediates JAK1 and JAK3 phosphorylation. In NKTCL, JAK3A572V and JAK3A573V mutations were identified in NK-S1 and MEC04 cell lines [67, 72]. These mutations were shown to trigger constitutive phosphorylation of JAK3, STAT3 [72], and STAT5 [67], respectively, in these cell lines and the ability of IL-2 to independently proliferate in cell culture [67].

4.2.3 JAK3M511I mutation in AML

AML is associated with different karyotype anomalies, and these aberrations are determinant of prognosis. An array-based analysis of human leukemia exemplars could identify the JAK3 M511I mutation [73]. It is located between the SH2 domain and the pseudokinase domain of JAK3. When JAK3M511I is introduced in 32D mouse cell line, which depends on interleukin-3 (IL-3) to grow, cells are able to survive in the absence of the cytokine and they do not differentiate in the presence of G-CSF [73]. Moreover, mice with hematopoietic stem cells infected with retrovirus encoding JAK3M511I showed a marked lymphocytosis in peripheral blood and spleen expansion, developing T-ALL [73, 74].

4.3 JAK1 mutations

Considering its important role in lymphopoiesis, JAK1-activating mutations have also been described in several lymphoid neoplasms, with highest frequency (7–27%) in T-ALL, but also in B-ALL and T cell prolymphocytic leukemia, and more rarely in ALL and AML [9]. Most of these mutations occur within the pseudokinase domain of JAK1. Certainly, the oncogenic potential of JAK1 pseudokinase domain disruption had been previously predicted since introduction of a V658F mutation in JAK1 (homologous to the V617F mutation in JAK2) led to its constitutive activation [75]. Recently, the mutation JAK1A634D was identified in adult T-ALL, and it was shown to lead to constitutive JAK1 activation when overexpressed in JAK1-deficient cell lines. Furthermore, A634D was shown to induce the autonomous growth of the cytokine-dependent Ba/F3 cell line, whereas it protected the murine ALL cell line BW5147 from dexamethasone-induced apoptosis. A recent study discovered another JAK1 mutation called JAK1S646P, showing that it is an activating mutation both *in vitro* and *in vivo* in ALL [76]. The first group in reporting somatic JAK1 mutations in AML (JAK1T478S and JAK1V623A) exposed that these mutations may function as disease-modifying mutations in AML, since they do not directly induce cell transformation, but rather modify the activation of downstream signaling pathways in response to external stimuli [77].

Fusion proteins	Disease
TEL-JAK2	T-ALL
BCD-JAK2	Atypical CML
PCM1-JAK2	AML, T-ALL
RPN1-JAK2	PMF
SSBP2-JAK2	B-ALL
PAX5-JAK2	B-ALL

Table 3.
Most common JAK2 fusion proteins in hematological cancer.

4.4 JAK fusion proteins

Historically, the identification of oncogenic fusion proteins involving JAK kinase domain entailed the first evidence of the key role of JAK kinases in HCs [31]. After this finding, acquired lesions involving JAK1, JAK2, and JAK3 (but not TYK2) have been reported in both AML and ALL. Interestingly, artificial chimeric TEL-JAK1, TEL-JAK3, and TEL-TYK2 proteins are able to sustain cytokine-independent growth in Ba/F3 cells [78] in which the expression of TEL-JAK2 protects Ba/F3 cells from IL-3 withdrawal-induced apoptotic cell death and leads to IL-3-independent growth. Furthermore, mice transplanted with bone marrow cells containing the ETV6-JAK2 fusion have been shown to develop leukemia [79]. There is no patient-derived chromosomal translocation that fuses the kinase domain of JAK1, JAK3, or TYK2 to a dimerizer described so far. This is probably related to an intrinsic genetic instability of the JAK2 locus, which can otherwise also be subject to amplifications in 30–50% of Hodgkin lymphomas and primary peripheral B-cell lymphomas [80–82]. The chromosomal translocation [t(9;12) (p24;p13)] is associated with T cell childhood ALL and results in the production of the fusion protein TEL-JAK2 (also known as ETV6-JAK2), which contains the JAK2 catalytic domain (JH1) and the oligomerization domain of TEL, one of the Ets transcription factor family members [31, 83]. The TEL subunit facilitates homodimerization of TEL-JAK2 molecules, thus facilitating transphosphorylation and activation of the JAK2 kinase domains. Several analogous JAK2 fusion proteins have since been described in ALLs or AMLs, including PCM1-JAK2 [84], BCR-JAK2 [85], RPN1-JAK2 [86], SSBP2-JAK2 [87], and PAX5-JAK2 [88] (**Table 3**). In all cases, the mechanism of JAK2 activation is thought to be similar, with the JAK2 fusion partner promoting dimerization and constitutive activation of the JAK2 tyrosine kinase component of the fusion protein, which constitutively triggers several downstream signal transduction pathways, such as STAT3, STAT5 [31, 89, 90], MAP kinase [91], PI3-kinase/Akt [92, 93], and NF-kB [94] independent of the presence of anchoring receptors.

5. JAK inhibitors and hematological cancer treatment

The starting point for the development of JAK inhibitors is located in 2005 when the JAK2V617F mutation was identified as the main cause of the majority of BCR-ABL1-negative myeloproliferative neoplasms (MPNs). Subsequently, the search for JAK inhibitors, and its development, continued with the discovery of other driver mutations (calreticulin (CALR) and myeloproliferative leukemia (MPL) virus oncogene) that also produce a constitutive JAK2 activation and, thus, aberrant JAK-STAT signaling [35, 36, 40, 95–97]. JAK inhibitors could be classified into different groups depending on their mechanism of action/region targeted in JAK: type I (they target the ATP-binding site of JAKs in the active conformation of the kinase domain), type II (they target the ATP-binding pocket of kinase domain in inactive conformation), and allosteric inhibitors (they bind to a different site from the ATP-binding site) [98]. All JAK inhibitors that have been clinically tested are type I, so this section of the present book chapter will focus on them.

5.1 Type I inhibitors

These compounds may be differentiated according to their specificity for each JAK. Most often they target JAK2, JAK1, and other kinases, such as TYK2 (e.g., ruxolitinib and momelotinib (CYT-387) or JAK3 and JAK1 (tofacitinib)). Some of them can inhibit all JAKs (e.g., gandotinib and peficitinib) and less frequently they specifically target JAK2 (e.g., pacritinib, NS-018 and CEP-33779), JAK1 (e.g., filgotinib and itacitinib) or JAK3 (e.g., decernotinib and JANEX 1) [98–100]. Type I JAK2 inhibitors are commonly used in MPNs, such as myelofibrosis (MF), polycythemia vera (PV), and essential thrombocythemia (ET) [101–104]. However, type I JAK inhibitors that target JAK1 and/or JAK3 are utilized to treat inflammation and autoimmune diseases [105]. Toxicity of type I inhibitors is also related to their specificity for the different JAKs: hematologic dyscrasia/immune suppression for JAK2 inhibitors [106] and immune suppression for JAK1 and JAK3 inhibitors [107]. At this point, it should be kept in mind that JAK2 cannot be completely long term inhibited because this will produce a severe cytopenia and even lead to aplastic anemia, since wild-type JAK2 (WT-JAK2) is indispensable for normal hematopoiesis. Thus, these inhibitors may be therapeutically used because they only partially inhibit JAK2 *in vivo*.

5.1.1 Ruxolitinib

Nowadays, ruxolitinib is the only type I JAK2 inhibitor that has been approved by the US Food and Drug Administration (FDA) to be used in the treatment of MF and hydroxyurea (HU)-resistant or HU-intolerant PVs [101, 108, 109]. Approval for MF was due to the two key phase 3 studies: Controlled Myelofibrosis study with Oral JAK inhibitor Treatment I and II (COMFORT-I and II) [108, 109]. In both studies, ruxolitinib was very effective in reducing spleen size and improving MF-general symptoms with dose-dependent anemia and thrombocytopenia, due to JAK2 inhibition, as the most frequent hematological side effect. However, anemia was well managed with dose adjustments and/or red blood cell transfusions [108]. Moreover, in both trials, ruxolitinib significantly reduced the risk of death [110]. In HU-refractory PVs, ruxolitinib effectively controls hematocrit, reduces spleen volume, and decreases JAK2V617F allele burden [101, 111]. Combined therapy with ruxolitinib and other JAK2 inhibitors may provide novel therapeutic strategies for the treatment of MPNs. Notably, it has been recently reported that combinations of ruxolitinib and vorinostat, a histone deacetylase (HDAC) inhibitor that down-regulates JAK2 expression, acted synergistically to reduce tumor growth in several hematological cancer cell lines (B cell lymphoma, multiple myeloma, anaplastic cell lymphoma, chronic B cell leukemia, and Hodgkin lymphoma) [112]. Moreover, this synergic effect on tumor cell growth was related to reduced glucose metabolism and induced ROS production and apoptosis [112]. These findings provide the rationale to support future clinical trials evaluating ruxolitinib-vorinostat combinations in patients. This combinatorial strategy has proved effective even in CML (BCR-ABL$^+$ myeloproliferative neoplasm). Thus, it has been shown that synergic combinations of ruxolitinib and nilotinib (a direct BCR-ABL inhibitor) profoundly inhibit JAK2 and STAT5 phosphorylation and induce apoptosis in primary CML CD34⁺ cells. These effects contribute to an effective elimination of these cells *in vitro* and *in vivo* and support the current utilization of ruxolitinib/nilotinib combinations in clinical trials to eradicate persistent disease in CML patients [113]. In fact, a phase I and a phase I/II clinical studies are already underway to evaluate the potential synergic effects of ruxolitinib-tyrosine kinase inhibitors combinations, such as nilotinib/imatinib, on eradicating CML stem/progenitor cells (ClinicalTrials.gov identifiers: NCT01702064 and NCT01751425).

5.1.2 Momelotinib

Given its potential clinical relevance, there are other type I JAK inhibitors that should be highlighted: momelotinib (CYT38) is a dual JAK1/2 inhibitor that, similar to ruxolitinib, reduces spleen size and MPN general related symptoms in intermediate or high-risk MF patients [114, 115]. Relevant, momelotinib has been shown to reduce anemia, which is a major issue in MF, so this drug might be an alternative to ruxolitinib for MPN patients with anemia. However, two phase-3 studies, SIMPLIFY-1 and SIMPLIFY-2, have reported that momelotinib does not seem to have major advantages over ruxolitinib, although it was related to less transfusion requirement [116, 117]. These findings have caused that momelotinib development has been stopped.

5.1.3 Pacritinib

Pacritinib (SB1518) is a JAK2-selective inhibitor (it does not inhibit JAK1) that also inhibits FLT3 (FMS-like tyrosine kinase 3, a key target in the therapeutics of acute myeloid leukemia), colony-stimulating factor 1 receptor (CSF1R) and interleukin-1 receptor-associated kinase 1 (IRAK1) [118]. In phase I/II studies, pacritinib, at a recommended dose of 400 mg/day, showed a good activity in MF patients with gastrointestinal alterations being the most frequent side effect [119, 120]. After these promising results, two phase-3 clinical trials (PERSIST 1 and 2) were initiated testing different pacritinib concentrations [121]. However, in 2016, FDA carried out a full clinical hold on these trials due to a suspected excess of mortality in treated patients caused by intracranial hemorrhage and cardiac events. This clinical hold was lifted by the FDA on January 2017 [121] and subsequently CTI Biopharma announced PAC203, a new trial in which different doses of pacritinib are being evaluated in MF patients with thrombocytopenia.

5.1.4 NS-108

NS-108 is a potent JAK2-selective inhibitor that also inhibits Src kinases [122]. This compound showed selectivity and high potency for JAK2V617F mutant in mouse models without producing anemia or thrombocytopenia [122]. NS-108 has been tested in a phase II trial at a recommended dose of 300 mg/day in MF patients. As previously described for other JAK2 inhibitors, NS-108 significantly reduced spleen size and improved general MF-related symptoms. However, this product was not able to significantly reduce the amount of JAK2V617F mutant cells [123].

5.1.5 Gandotinib

Gandotinib (LY2784544) is a selective and potent inhibitor of JAK2V617F [124]. This drug has been evaluated in a phase I trial for safety, tolerability, and pharmacokinetic parameters in patients with MF, PV, and ET. Treatment with this compound at 120 mg/day (oral recommended phase II dose) was associated with an acceptable safety/tolerability and with clinical improvements in MPN JAK2V617F patients [103]. These findings provide rationale for further gandotinib clinical testing.

5.2 Type II inhibitors

Two type II JAK2 inhibitors (NVP-BBT594 and NVP-CHZ868) have been developed. NVP-BBT594 was effective in MPN cellular models [125] and NVP-CHZ868 in preclinical mouse MPN models. However, JAK2 inhibition caused by type II inhibitors is more effective and powerful than that produced by type I inhibitors, which in turn may induce profound cytopenia, limiting its future development and clinical use.

5.3 Allosteric inhibitors

In this group are the so-called type III (they bind to a site close to the ATP-binding site, e.g., LS104 [126]) and type IV inhibitors (they bind to an allosteric site distant from the ATP-binding site, e.g., ON044580 [127]). Since these inhibitors do not target the ATP pocket, hypothetically, they are more specific than type I/II JAK inhibitors due to the high homology shown by the ATP-binding sites. Taking this into account, JAK allosteric inhibitors would be particularly indicated to treat MPNs related to JAK mutations (especially JAK2V617F) as an efficient inhibition of WT-JAK2 will always produce a profound cytopenia. Nowadays, there is no a JAK allosteric inhibitor in clinical development.

6. Conclusions

In summary, JAK kinases are key proteins in the development of hematological malignancies, since different genetic alterations including fusion protein formation, gene amplification, and point mutations have been discovered in a wide array of hematological malignancies. Particularly, JAK somatic point mutations have been detected in a high proportion of HC patients. Furthermore, detection of JAK mutations is beginning to provide prognostic information. For all these reasons, manipulating JAK activity currently constitutes an interesting therapeutic strategy and an interesting biomarker in hematological cancer. A great effort has been made by researchers in the last decade to find and characterize novel JAK inhibitors that might be clinically used, and, in fact, some of them have already reached clinical evaluation. However, more efforts are needed in order to identify more JAK mutations that lead to develop more accurate therapies against specific malignancies.

Acknowledgements

We thank all the authors who contributed to the understanding of the cross-talk between the JAK kinase and hematological cancer. We apologize to those whose work deserves to be cited but unfortunately are not quoted because of space restriction. The research program in the author's lab was supported by grants-in-aid from the Spanish Ministry of Economy and Competitivity (MINECO) with the funding of European Regional Development Fund-European Social Fund (SAF2015-65113-C2-2-R), and Alfredo Martin-Reyes Foundation (Arehucas)-FICIC. CR and MMG were supported by postdoctoral grants-in-aid from the MINECO-Juan de la Cierva Program and ULPGC, respectively.

Conflict of interest

The authors declare that the research was conducted in the absence of any commercial or financial relationships that could be construed as a potential conflict of interest.

Author details

Carlota Recio*, Haidée Aranda-Tavío, Miguel Guerra-Rodríguez, Mercedes de Mirecki-Garrido, Patricia Martín-Rodríguez, Borja Guerra and Leandro Fernández-Pérez
Institute for Research in Biomedicine and Health (IUIBS), University of Las Palmas de Gran Canaria (ULPGC), Las Palmas de Gran Canaria, Spain

*Address all correspondence to: carlota.recio@ulpgc.es

References

[1] O'Shea JJ, Schwartz DM, Villarino AV, Gadina M, McInnes IB, Laurence A. The JAK-STAT pathway: Impact on human disease and therapeutic intervention. Annual Review of Medicine. 2015;**66**:311-328

[2] Levy DE, Darnell JE. Stats: Transcriptional control and biological impact. Nature Reviews. Molecular Cell Biology. 2002;**3**(9):651-662

[3] Leonard WJ, O'Shea JJ. Jaks and STATs: Biological implications. Annual Review of Immunology. 1998;**16**:293-322

[4] Harrison DA. The Jak/STAT pathway. Cold Spring Harbor Perspectives in Biology. 2012;**4**:a011205

[5] Ghoreschi K, Laurence A, O'Shea JJ. Janus kinases in immune cell signaling. Immunological Reviews. 2009;**228**(1):273-287

[6] Kiu H, Nicholson SE. Biology and significance of the JAK/STAT signalling pathways. Growth Factors. 2012;**30**(2):88-106

[7] Miklossy G, Hilliard TS, Turkson J. Therapeutic modulators of STAT signalling for human diseases. Nature Reviews. Drug Discovery. 2013;**12**(8):611-629

[8] Senkevitch E, Durum S. The promise of Janus kinase inhibitors in the treatment of hematological malignancies. Cytokine. 2017;**98**:33-41

[9] Springuel L, Renauld JC, Knoops L. JAK kinase targeting in hematologic malignancies: A sinuous pathway from identification of genetic alterations towards clinical indications. Haematologica. 2015;**100**(10):1240-1253

[10] Yamaoka K. Janus kinase inhibitors for rheumatoid arthritis. Current Opinion in Chemical Biology. 2016;**32**:29-33

[11] Banerjee S, Biehl A, Gadina M, Hasni S, Schwartz DM. JAK-STAT signaling as a target for inflammatory and autoimmune diseases: Current and future prospects. Drugs. 2017;**77**(5):521-546

[12] Vainchenker W, Dusa A, Constantinescu SN. JAKs in pathology: Role of Janus kinases in hematopoietic malignancies and immunodeficiencies. Seminars in Cell & Developmental Biology. 2008;**19**(4):385-393

[13] Schindler C, Levy DE, Decker T. JAK-STAT signaling: From interferons to cytokines. The Journal of Biological Chemistry. 2007;**282**(28):20059-20063

[14] Ehret GB, Reichenbach P, Schindler U, Horvath CM, Fritz S, Nabholz M, et al. DNA binding specificity of different STAT proteins. Comparison of in vitro specificity with natural target sites. The Journal of Biological Chemistry. 2001;**276**(9):6675-6688

[15] Stark GR, Darnell JE. The JAK-STAT pathway at twenty. Immunity. 2012;**36**(4):503-514

[16] Schindler C, Plumlee C. Inteferons pen the JAK-STAT pathway. Seminars in Cell & Developmental Biology. 2008;**19**(4):311-318

[17] Seidel HM, Lamb P, Rosen J. Pharmaceutical intervention in the JAK/STAT signaling pathway. Oncogene. 2000;**19**(21):2645-2656

[18] Haura EB, Turkson J, Jove R. Mechanisms of disease: Insights into the emerging role of signal transducers and activators of transcription in cancer. Nature Clinical Practice. Oncology. 2005;**2**(6):315-324

[19] Braunstein J, Brutsaert S, Olson R, Schindler C. STATs dimerize in the absence of phosphorylation. The

Journal of Biological Chemistry. 2003;**278**(36):34133-34140

[20] Dawson MA, Bannister AJ, Göttgens B, Foster SD, Bartke T, Green AR, et al. JAK2 phosphorylates histone H3Y41 and excludes HP1alpha from chromatin. Nature. 2009;**461**(7265):819-822

[21] Yang S, Park K, Turkson J, Arteaga CL. Ligand-independent phosphorylation of Y869 (Y845) links mutant EGFR signaling to stat-mediated gene expression. Experimental Cell Research. 2008;**314**(2):413-419

[22] Hu X, Dutta P, Tsurumi A, Li J, Wang J, Land H, et al. Unphosphorylated STAT5A stabilizes heterochromatin and suppresses tumor growth. Proceedings of the National Academy of Sciences of the United States of America. 2013;**110**(25):10213-10218

[23] Shuai K, Liu B. Regulation of JAK-STAT signalling in the immune system. Nature Reviews. Immunology. 2003;**3**(11):900-911

[24] Espert L, Dusanter-Fourt I, Chelbi-Alix MK. [Negative regulation of the JAK/STAT: Pathway implication in tumorigenesis]. Bulletin du Cancer. 2005;**92**(10):845-857

[25] Larsen L, Röpke C. Suppressors of cytokine signalling: SOCS. APMIS. 2002;**110**(12):833-844

[26] Trengove MC, Ward AC. SOCS proteins in development and disease. American Journal of Clinical and Experimental Immunology. 2013;**2**(1):1-29

[27] Ward AC, Touw I, Yoshimura A. The Jak-Stat pathway in normal and perturbed hematopoiesis. Blood. 2000;**95**(1):19-29

[28] Bromberg J. Stat proteins and oncogenesis. The Journal of Clinical Investigation. 2002;**109**(9):1139-1142

[29] Groner B, Hennighausen L. The versatile regulation of cellular events by Jak-Stat signaling: From transcriptional control to microtubule dynamics and energy metabolism. Hormone Molecular Biology and Clinical Investigation. 2012;**10**(1):193-200

[30] Rani A, Murphy JJ. STAT5 in cancer and immunity. Journal of Interferon & Cytokine Research. 2016;**36**(4):226-237

[31] Lacronique V, Boureux A, Valle VD, Poirel H, Quang CT, Mauchauffé M, et al. A TEL-JAK2 fusion protein with constitutive kinase activity in human leukemia. Science. 1997;**278**(5341):1309-1312

[32] Hammarén HM, Virtanen AT, Raivola J, Silvennoinen O. The regulation of JAKs in cytokine signaling and its breakdown in disease. Cytokine. 2018;pii:S1043-4666 (18) 30127-3

[33] Constantinescu SN, Girardot M, Pecquet C. Mining for JAK-STAT mutations in cancer. Trends in Biochemical Sciences. 2008;**33**(3):122-131

[34] Vardiman JW, Harris NL, Brunning RD. The World Health Organization (WHO) classification of the myeloid neoplasms. Blood. 2002;**100**(7):2292-2302

[35] Baxter EJ, Scott LM, Campbell PJ, East C, Fourouclas N, Swanton S, et al. Acquired mutation of the tyrosine kinase JAK2 in human myeloproliferative disorders. Lancet. 2005;**365**(9464):1054-1061

[36] James C, Ugo V, Le Couédic JP, Staerk J, Delhommeau F, Lacout C, et al. A unique clonal JAK2 mutation leading to constitutive signalling causes polycythaemia vera. Nature. 2005;**434**(7037):1144-1148

[37] Zhao R, Xing S, Li Z, Fu X, Li Q, Krantz SB, et al. Identification of an acquired JAK2 mutation

in polycythemia vera. The Journal of Biological Chemistry. 2005;**280**(24):22788-22792

[38] Butcher CM, Hahn U, To LB, Gecz J, Wilkins EJ, Scott HS, et al. Two novel JAK2 exon 12 mutations in JAK2V617F-negative polycythaemia vera patients. Leukemia. 2008;**22**(4):870-873

[39] Saeidi K. Myeloproliferative neoplasms: Current molecular biology and genetics. Critical Reviews in Oncology/Hematology. 2016;**98**:375-389

[40] Kralovics R, Passamonti F, Buser AS, Teo SS, Tiedt R, Passweg JR, et al. A gain-of-function mutation of JAK2 in myeloproliferative disorders. The New England Journal of Medicine. 2005;**352**(17):1779-1790

[41] Larsen TS, Christensen JH, Hasselbalch HC, Pallisgaard N. The JAK2 V617F mutation involves B- and T-lymphocyte lineages in a subgroup of patients with Philadelphia-chromosome negative chronic myeloproliferative disorders. British Journal of Haematology. 2007;**136**(5):745-751

[42] Morgan KJ, Gilliland DG. A role for JAK2 mutations in myeloproliferative diseases. Annual Review of Medicine. 2008;**59**:213-222

[43] O'Shea JJ, Holland SM, Staudt LM. JAKs and STATs in immunity, immunodeficiency, and cancer. The New England Journal of Medicine. 2013;**368**(2):161-170

[44] Van Etten RA. Aberrant cytokine signaling in leukemia. Oncogene. 2007;**26**(47):6738-6749

[45] Levine RL, Gilliland DG. JAK-2 mutations and their relevance to myeloproliferative disease. Current Opinion in Hematology. 2007;**14**(1):43-47

[46] Lu X, Levine R, Tong W, Wernig G, Pikman Y, Zarnegar S, et al. Expression of a homodimeric type I cytokine receptor is required for JAK2V617F-mediated transformation. Proceedings of the National Academy of Sciences of the United States of America. 2005;**102**(52):18962-18967

[47] Lacout C, Pisani DF, Tulliez M, Gachelin FM, Vainchenker W, Villeval JL. JAK2V617F expression in murine hematopoietic cells leads to MPD mimicking human PV with secondary myelofibrosis. Blood. 2006;**108**(5):1652-1660

[48] Funakoshi-Tago M, Pelletier S, Matsuda T, Parganas E, Ihle JN. Receptor specific downregulation of cytokine signaling by autophosphorylation in the FERM domain of Jak2. The EMBO Journal. 2006;**25**(20):4763-4772

[49] Teofili L, Martini M, Cenci T, Petrucci G, Torti L, Storti S, et al. Different STAT-3 and STAT-5 phosphorylation discriminates among Ph-negative chronic myeloproliferative diseases and is independent of the V617F JAK-2 mutation. Blood. 2007;**110**(1):354-359

[50] Colaizzo D, Amitrano L, Tiscia GL, Grandone E, Guardascione MA, Margaglione M. A new JAK2 gene mutation in patients with polycythemia vera and splanchnic vein thrombosis. Blood. 2007;**110**(7):2768-2769

[51] Pardanani A, Lasho TL, Finke C, Hanson CA, Tefferi A. Prevalence and clinicopathologic correlates of JAK2 exon 12 mutations in JAK2V617F-negative polycythemia vera. Leukemia. 2007;**21**(9):1960-1963

[52] Williams DM, Kim AH, Rogers O, Spivak JL, Moliterno AR. Phenotypic variations and new mutations in JAK2 V617F-negative polycythemia vera, erythrocytosis, and idiopathic myelofibrosis. Experimental Hematology. 2007;**35**(11):1641-1646

[53] Scott LM, Tong W, Levine RL, Scott MA, Beer PA, Stratton MR, et al. JAK2 exon 12 mutations in polycythemia vera and idiopathic erythrocytosis. The New England Journal of Medicine. 2007;**356**(5):459-468

[54] Pietra D, Li S, Brisci A, Passamonti F, Rumi E, Theocharides A, et al. Somatic mutations of JAK2 exon 12 in patients with JAK2 (V617F)-negative myeloproliferative disorders. Blood. 2008;**111**(3):1686-1689

[55] Hahn AW, Li B, Prouet P, Giri S, Pathak R, Martin MG. Acute megakaryocytic leukemia: What have we learned. Blood Reviews. 2016;**30**(1):49-53

[56] Mercher T, Wernig G, Moore SA, Levine RL, Gu T-L, Fröhling S, et al. JAK2T875N is a novel activating mutation that results in myeloproliferative disease with features of megakaryoblastic leukemia in a murine bone marrow transplantation model. Blood. 2006;**108**(8):2770-2779

[57] Hitzler JK, Cheung J, Li Y, Scherer SW, Zipursky A. GATA1 mutations in transient leukemia and acute megakaryoblastic leukemia of Down syndrome. Blood. 2003;**101**(11):4301-4304

[58] Mercher T, Coniat MB, Monni R, Mauchauffe M, Nguyen Khac F, Gressin L, et al. Involvement of a human gene related to the Drosophila spen gene in the recurrent t(1;22) translocation of acute megakaryocytic leukemia. Proceedings of the National Academy of Sciences of the United States of America. 2001;**98**(10):5776-5779

[59] Li Z, Godinho FJ, Klusmann J-H, Garriga-Canut M, Yu C, Orkin SH. Developmental stage–selective effect of somatically mutated leukemogenic transcription factor GATA1. Nature Genetics. 2005;**37**:613

[60] Zou H, Yan D, Mohi G. Differential biological activity of disease-associated JAK2 mutants. FEBS Letters. 2011;**585**(7):1007-1013

[61] Haan S, Wuller S, Kaczor J, Rolvering C, Nocker T, Behrmann I, et al. SOCS-mediated downregulation of mutant Jak2 (V617F, T875N and K539L) counteracts cytokine-independent signaling. Oncogene. 2009;**28**(34):3069-3080

[62] Lee P, Bhansali R, Izraeli S, Hijiya N, Crispino JD. The biology, pathogenesis and clinical aspects of acute lymphoblastic leukemia in children with Down syndrome. Leukemia. 2016;**30**(9):1816-1823

[63] Bercovich D, Ganmore I, Scott LM, Wainreb G, Birger Y, Elimelech A, et al. Mutations of JAK2 in acute lymphoblastic leukaemias associated with Down's syndrome. Lancet. 2008;**372**(9648):1484-1492

[64] Malinge S, Ben-Abdelali R, Settegrana C, Radford-Weiss I, Debre M, Beldjord K, et al. Novel activating JAK2 mutation in a patient with Down syndrome and B-cell precursor acute lymphoblastic leukemia. Blood. 2007;**109**(5):2202-2204

[65] Tomoyasu C, Imamura T, Tomii T, Yano M, Asai D, Goto H, et al. Copy number abnormality of acute lymphoblastic leukemia cell lines based on their genetic subtypes. International Journal of Hematology. 2018;**108**(3):312-318

[66] Cornejo MG, Kharas MG, Werneck MB, Le Bras S, Moore SA, Ball B, et al. Constitutive JAK3 activation induces lymphoproliferative syndromes in murine bone marrow transplantation models. Blood. 2009;**113**(12):2746-2754

[67] Koo GC, Tan SY, Tang T, Poon SL, Allen GE, Tan L, et al. Janus kinase 3-activating mutations identified in

natural killer/T-cell lymphoma. Cancer Discovery. 2012;**2**(7):591-597

[68] Bellanger D, Jacquemin V, Chopin M, Pierron G, Bernard OA, Ghysdael J, et al. Recurrent JAK1 and JAK3 somatic mutations in T-cell prolymphocytic leukemia. Leukemia. 2014;**28**(2):417-419

[69] Russell SM, Tayebi N, Nakajima H, Riedy MC, Roberts JL, Aman MJ, et al. Mutation of Jak3 in a patient with SCID: Essential role of Jak3 in lymphoid development. Science. 1995;**270**(5237):797-800

[70] Walters DK, Mercher T, Gu TL, O' Hare T, Tyner JW, Loriaux M, et al. Activating alleles of JAK3 in acute megakaryoblastic leukemia. Cancer Cell. 2006;**10**(1):65-75

[71] Malinge S, Ragu C, Della-Valle V, Pisani D, Constantinescu SN, Perez C, et al. Activating mutations in human acute megakaryoblastic leukemia. Blood. 2008;**112**(10):4220-4226

[72] Bouchekioua A, Scourzic L, de Wever O, Zhang Y, Cervera P, Aline-Fardin A, et al. JAK3 deregulation by activating mutations confers invasive growth advantage in extranodal nasal-type natural killer cell lymphoma. Leukemia. 2014;**28**(2):338-348

[73] Yamashita Y, Yuan J, Suetake I, Suzuki H, Ishikawa Y, Choi YL, et al. Array-based genomic resequencing of human leukemia. Oncogene. 2010;**29**(25):3723-3731

[74] Degryse S, Bornschein S, de Bock CE, Leroy E, Vanden Bempt M, Demeyer S, et al. Mutant JAK3 signaling is increased by loss of wild-type JAK3 or by acquisition of secondary JAK3 mutations in T-ALL. Blood. 2018;**131**(4):421-425

[75] Chen E, Staudt LM, Green AR. Janus kinase deregulation in leukemia and lymphoma. Immunity. 2012;**36**(4):529-541

[76] Li Q, Li B, Hu L, Ning H, Jiang M, Wang D, et al. Identification of a novel functional JAK1 S646P mutation in acute lymphoblastic leukemia. Oncotarget. 2017;**8**(21):34687-34697

[77] Xiang Z, Zhao Y, Mitaksov V, Fremont DH, Kasai Y, Molitoris A, et al. Identification of somatic JAK1 mutations in patients with acute myeloid leukemia. Blood. 2008;**111**(9):4809-4812

[78] Lacronique V, Boureux A, Monni R, Dumon S, Mauchauffe M, Mayeux P, et al. Transforming properties of chimeric TEL-JAK proteins in Ba/F3 cells. Blood. 2000;**95**(6):2076-2083

[79] Schwaller J, Frantsve J, Aster J, Williams IR, Tomasson MH, Ross TS, et al. Transformation of hematopoietic cell lines to growth-factor independence and induction of a fatal myelo- and lymphoproliferative disease in mice by retrovirally transduced TEL/JAK2 fusion genes. The EMBO Journal. 1998;**17**(18):5321-5333

[80] Joos S, Kupper M, Ohl S, von Bonin F, Mechtersheimer G, Bentz M, et al. Genomic imbalances including amplification of the tyrosine kinase gene JAK2 in CD30+ Hodgkin cells. Cancer Research. 2000;**60**(3):549-552

[81] Rosenwald A, Wright G, Leroy K, Yu X, Gaulard P, Gascoyne RD, et al. Molecular diagnosis of primary mediastinal B cell lymphoma identifies a clinically favorable subgroup of diffuse large B cell lymphoma related to Hodgkin lymphoma. The Journal of Experimental Medicine. 2003;**198**(6):851-862

[82] Lenz G, Wright GW, Emre NC, Kohlhammer H, Dave SS, Davis RE, et al. Molecular subtypes of diffuse large B-cell lymphoma arise by distinct

genetic pathways. Proceedings of the National Academy of Sciences of the United States of America. 2008;**105**(36):13520-13525

[83] Peeters P, Raynaud SD, Cools J, Wlodarska I, Grosgeorge J, Philip P, et al. Fusion of TEL, the ETS-variant gene 6 (ETV6), to the receptor-associated kinase JAK2 as a result of t(9;12) in a lymphoid and t(9;15;12) in a myeloid leukemia. Blood. 1997;**90**(7):2535-2540

[84] Reiter A, Walz C, Watmore A, Schoch C, Blau I, Schlegelberger B, et al. The t(8;9)(p22;p24) is a recurrent abnormality in chronic and acute leukemia that fuses PCM1 to JAK2. Cancer Research. 2005;**65**(7):2662-2667

[85] Griesinger F, Hennig H, Hillmer F, Podleschny M, Steffens R, Pies A, et al. A BCR-JAK2 fusion gene as the result of a t(9;22)(p24;q11.2) translocation in a patient with a clinically typical chronic myeloid leukemia. Genes, Chromosomes & Cancer. 2005;**44**(3):329-333

[86] Mark HF, Sotomayor EA, Nelson M, Chaves F, Sanger WG, Kaleem Z, et al. Chronic idiopathic myelofibrosis (CIMF) resulting from a unique 3;9 translocation disrupting the janus kinase 2 (JAK2) gene. Experimental and Molecular Pathology. 2006;**81**(3):217-223

[87] Poitras JL, Dal Cin P, Aster JC, Deangelo DJ, Morton CC. Novel SSBP2-JAK2 fusion gene resulting from a t(5;9)(q14.1;p24.1) in pre-B acute lymphocytic leukemia. Genes, Chromosomes & Cancer. 2008;**47**(10):884-889

[88] Nebral K, Denk D, Attarbaschi A, Konig M, Mann G, Haas OA, et al. Incidence and diversity of PAX5 fusion genes in childhood acute lymphoblastic leukemia. Leukemia. 2009;**23**(1):134-143

[89] Ho JM, Beattie BK, Squire JA, Frank DA, Barber DL. Fusion of the ets transcription factor TEL to Jak2 results in constitutive Jak-Stat signaling. Blood. 1999;**93**(12):4354-4364

[90] Carron C, Cormier F, Janin A, Lacronique V, Giovannini M, Daniel MT, et al. TEL-JAK2 transgenic mice develop T-cell leukemia. Blood. 2000;**95**(12):3891-3899

[91] Ho JM, Nguyen MH, Dierov JK, Badger KM, Beattie BK, Tartaro P, et al. TEL-JAK2 constitutively activates the extracellular signal-regulated kinase (ERK), stress-activated protein/Jun kinase (SAPK/JNK), and p38 signaling pathways. Blood. 2002;**100**(4):1438-1448

[92] Nguyen MH, Ho JM, Beattie BK, Barber DL. TEL-JAK2 mediates constitutive activation of the phosphatidylinositol 3′-kinase/protein kinase B signaling pathway. The Journal of Biological Chemistry. 2001;**276**(35):32704-32713

[93] Santos SC, Lacronique V, Bouchaert I, Monni R, Bernard O, Gisselbrecht S, et al. Constitutively active STAT5 variants induce growth and survival of hematopoietic cells through a PI 3-kinase/Akt dependent pathway. Oncogene. 2001;**20**(17):2080-2090

[94] Malinge S, Monni R, Bernard O, Penard-Lacronique V. Activation of the NF-kappaB pathway by the leukemogenic TEL-Jak2 and TEL-Abl fusion proteins leads to the accumulation of antiapoptotic IAP proteins and involves IKKalpha. Oncogene. 2006;**25**(25):3589-3597

[95] Arber DA, Orazi A, Hasserjian R, Thiele J, Borowitz MJ, Le Beau MM, et al. The 2016 revision to the World Health Organization classification of myeloid neoplasms and acute leukemia. Blood. 2016;**127**(20):2391-2405

[96] Levine RL, Wadleigh M, Cools J, Ebert BL, Wernig G, Huntly BJ, et al. Activating mutation in the tyrosine kinase JAK2 in polycythemia vera, essential thrombocythemia, and myeloid metaplasia with myelofibrosis. Cancer Cell. 2005;7(4):387-397

[97] Rampal R, Al-Shahrour F, Abdel-Wahab O, Patel JP, Brunel JP, Mermel CH, et al. Integrated genomic analysis illustrates the central role of JAK-STAT pathway activation in myeloproliferative neoplasm pathogenesis. Blood. 2014;**123**(22):e123-e133

[98] Vainchenker W, Leroy E, Gilles L, Marty C, Plo I, Constantinescu SN. JAK inhibitors for the treatment of myeloproliferative neoplasms and other disorders. F1000Res. 2018;7:82

[99] Bose P, Verstovsek S. Developmental therapeutics in myeloproliferative neoplasms. Clinical Lymphoma, Myeloma & Leukemia. 2017;**17S**:S43-S52

[100] Griesshammer M, Sadjadian P. The BCR-ABL1-negative myeloproliferative neoplasms: A review of JAK inhibitors in the therapeutic armamentarium. Expert Opinion on Pharmacotherapy. 2017;**18**(18):1929-1938

[101] Vannucchi AM, Kiladjian JJ, Griesshammer M, Masszi T, Durrant S, Passamonti F, et al. Ruxolitinib versus standard therapy for the treatment of polycythemia vera. The New England Journal of Medicine. 2015;**372**(5):426-435

[102] Pieri L, Pancrazzi A, Pacilli A, Rabuzzi C, Rotunno G, Fanelli T, et al. JAK2V617F complete molecular remission in polycythemia vera/essential thrombocythemia patients treated with ruxolitinib. Blood. 2015;**125**(21):3352-3353

[103] Verstovsek S, Mesa RA, Salama ME, Li L, Pitou C, Nunes FP, et al. A phase 1 study of the Janus kinase 2 (JAK2)(V617F) inhibitor, gandotinib (LY2784544), in patients with primary myelofibrosis, polycythemia vera, and essential thrombocythemia. Leukemia Research. 2017;**61**:89-95

[104] Verstovsek S, Courby S, Griesshammer M, Mesa RA, Brachmann CB, Kawashima J, et al. A phase 2 study of momelotinib, a potent JAK1 and JAK2 inhibitor, in patients with polycythemia vera or essential thrombocythemia. Leukemia Research. 2017;**60**:11-17

[105] Schwartz DM, Bonelli M, Gadina M, O'Shea JJ. Type I/II cytokines, JAKs, and new strategies for treating autoimmune diseases. Nature Reviews Rheumatology. 2016;**12**(1):25-36

[106] Tam CS, Kantarjian H, Cortes J, Lynn A, Pierce S, Zhou L, et al. Dynamic model for predicting death within 12 months in patients with primary or post-polycythemia vera/essential thrombocythemia myelofibrosis. Journal of Clinical Oncology. 2009;**27**(33):5587-5593

[107] Kleppe M, Spitzer MH, Li S, Hill CE, Dong L, Papalexi E, et al. Jak1 integrates cytokine sensing to regulate hematopoietic stem cell function and stress hematopoiesis. Cell Stem Cell. 2017;**21**(4):489-501 e7

[108] Harrison C, Kiladjian JJ, Al-Ali HK, Gisslinger H, Waltzman R, Stalbovskaya V, et al. JAK inhibition with ruxolitinib versus best available therapy for myelofibrosis. The New England Journal of Medicine. 2012;**366**(9):787-798

[109] Verstovsek S, Mesa RA, Gotlib J, Levy RS, Gupta V, DiPersio JF, et al. A double-blind, placebo-controlled trial of ruxolitinib for myelofibrosis. The New England Journal of Medicine. 2012;**366**(9):799-807

[110] Vannucchi AM, Kantarjian HM, Kiladjian JJ, Gotlib J, Cervantes F, Mesa RA, et al. A pooled analysis of

overall survival in COMFORT-I and COMFORT-II, 2 randomized phase III trials of ruxolitinib for the treatment of myelofibrosis. Haematologica. 2015;**100**(9):1139-1145

[111] Passamonti F, Griesshammer M, Palandri F, Egyed M, Benevolo G, Devos T, et al. Ruxolitinib for the treatment of inadequately controlled polycythaemia vera without splenomegaly (RESPONSE-2): A randomised, open-label, phase 3b study. The Lancet Oncology. 2017;**18**(1):88-99

[112] Civallero M, Cosenza M, Pozzi S, Sacchi S. Ruxolitinib combined with vorinostat suppresses tumor growth and alters metabolic phenotype in hematological diseases. Oncotarget. 2017;**8**(61):103797-103814

[113] Gallipoli P, Cook A, Rhodes S, Hopcroft L, Wheadon H, Whetton AD, et al. JAK2/STAT5 inhibition by nilotinib with ruxolitinib contributes to the elimination of CML CD34+ cells in vitro and in vivo. Blood. 2014;**124**(9):1492-1501

[114] Tefferi A, Barraco D, Lasho TL, Shah S, Begna KH, Al-Kali A, et al. Momelotinib therapy for myelofibrosis: A 7-year follow-up. Blood Cancer Journal. 2018;**8**(3):29

[115] Pardanani A, Gotlib J, Roberts AW, Wadleigh M, Sirhan S, Kawashima J, et al. Long-term efficacy and safety of momelotinib, a JAK1 and JAK2 inhibitor, for the treatment of myelofibrosis. Leukemia. 2018;**32**(4):1035-1038

[116] Mesa RA, Kiladjian JJ, Catalano JV, Devos T, Egyed M, Hellmann A, et al. SIMPLIFY-1: A phase III randomized trial of momelotinib versus ruxolitinib in janus kinase inhibitor-naive patients with myelofibrosis. Journal of Clinical Oncology. 2017;**35**(34):3844-3850

[117] Harrison CN, Vannucchi AM, Platzbecker U, Cervantes F, Gupta V, Lavie D, et al. Momelotinib versus best available therapy in patients with myelofibrosis previously treated with ruxolitinib (SIMPLIFY 2): A randomised, open-label, phase 3 trial. Lancet Haematology. 2018;**5**(2):e73-e81

[118] Poulsen A, William A, Blanchard S, Lee A, Nagaraj H, Wang H, et al. Structure-based design of oxygen-linked macrocyclic kinase inhibitors: Discovery of SB1518 and SB1578, potent inhibitors of Janus kinase 2 (JAK2) and Fms-like tyrosine kinase-3 (FLT3). Journal of Computer-Aided Molecular Design. 2012;**26**(4):437-450

[119] Verstovsek S, Odenike O, Singer JW, Granston T, Al-Fayoumi S, Deeg HJ. Phase 1/2 study of pacritinib, a next generation JAK2/FLT3 inhibitor, in myelofibrosis or other myeloid malignancies. Journal of Hematology & Oncology. 2016;**9**(1):137

[120] Komrokji RS, Seymour JF, Roberts AW, Wadleigh M, To LB, Scherber R, et al. Results of a phase 2 study of pacritinib (SB1518), a JAK2/JAK2(V617F) inhibitor, in patients with myelofibrosis. Blood. 2015;**125**(17):2649-2655

[121] Mesa RA, Vannucchi AM, Mead A, Egyed M, Szoke A, Suvorov A, et al. Pacritinib versus best available therapy for the treatment of myelofibrosis irrespective of baseline cytopenias (PERSIST-1): An international, randomised, phase 3 trial. Lancet Haematology. 2017;**4**(5):e225-ee36

[122] Nakaya Y, Shide K, Naito H, Niwa T, Horio T, Miyake J, et al. Effect of NS-018, a selective JAK2V617F inhibitor, in a murine model of myelofibrosis. Blood Cancer Journal. 2014;**4**:e174

[123] Verstovsek S, Talpaz M, Ritchie E, Wadleigh M, Odenike O, Jamieson C, et al. A phase I, open-label, dose-escalation, multicenter study of the JAK2 inhibitor NS-018 in patients

with myelofibrosis. Leukemia. 2017;**31**(2):393-402

[124] Ma L, Clayton JR, Walgren RA, Zhao B, Evans RJ, Smith MC, et al. Discovery and characterization of LY2784544, a small-molecule tyrosine kinase inhibitor of JAK2V617F. Blood Cancer Journal. 2013;**3**:e109

[125] Andraos R, Qian Z, Bonenfant D, Rubert J, Vangrevelinghe E, Scheufler C, et al. Modulation of activation-loop phosphorylation by JAK inhibitors is binding mode dependent. Cancer Discovery. 2012;**2**(6):512-523

[126] Lipka DB, Hoffmann LS, Heidel F, Markova B, Blum MC, Breitenbuecher F, et al. LS104, a non-ATP-competitive small-molecule inhibitor of JAK2, is potently inducing apoptosis in JAK2V617F-positive cells. Molecular Cancer Therapeutics. 2008;7(5):1176-1184

[127] Jatiani SS, Cosenza SC, Reddy MV, Ha JH, Baker SJ, Samanta AK, et al. A non-ATP-competitive dual inhibitor of JAK2 and BCR-ABL kinases: Elucidation of a novel therapeutic spectrum based on substrate competitive inhibition. Genes & Cancer. 2010;**1**(4):331-345

Section 3

Cancer Treatment by Tyrosine Kinase Inhibitors

Chapter 4

Noncoding RNAs as Predictive Biomarkers of Therapeutic Response to Tyrosine Kinase Inhibitors in Metastatic Cancer

Julia Kovacova and Ondrej Slaby

Abstract

Since their discovery, noncoding RNAs have acquired extensive attention due to their eminent role in the regulation of gene expression and thus also in the pathogenesis of many diseases. Currently, strong evidence is showing that noncoding RNAs are integral parts of key cancer-related cellular pathways, and the deregulation of their levels is pathogenetic on one hand but feasible as a biomarker of pathogenesis itself on the other hand. In cancer, diagnosis, prognosis, and prediction of therapy outcome can be derived from levels of various noncoding RNAs. This chapter is focused on potential application of noncoding RNAs in prediction of therapeutic response to tyrosine kinase inhibitors commonly used as targeted therapy in a wide range of metastatic cancers.

Keywords: biomarker, response, ncRNA, tyrosine kinase inhibitors

1. Introduction

Since the 1980s there was some spare evidence of low-molecular RNAs being able to bind complementarily to bigger RNA molecules and having a role in chromatin organization. Small nuclear RNAs (snRNAs) and small nucleolar RNAs (snoRNAs) [1–4] were the early discoveries in noncoding RNA field besides tRNAs, and at first, it looked like an exotic exception in rather binary world of protein-coding sequences and the rest of the genome which considered to be "junk" DNA. At the time some mechanisms of regulation of gene expression were known, and overall picture seemed to be complete, give or take a few details. Although it was known that mRNA is a vital part of gene expression and central dogma of molecular biology, the only functional product arising from genetic information, as it was commonly believed, is protein. As the genomic era was just about to come, there was no reason to think that most RNA transcripts are not translated.

Such remarks were first made in 1995 with H19. Expression of this lncRNA correlated with bladder carcinoma caused by loss of H19 imprinting pattern [5]. Further evidence was provided after discovery of other noncoding transcripts, for example, growth arrest-specific 5 (GAS5) [6] and, most importantly, prostate cancer antigen 3 (PCA3/DD3) highly overexpressed in prostate tumor tissue [7].

The beginning of the millennium was marked by the discovery of RNA interference and new short noncoding RNAs regulating gene expression and thus developmental timing in *Caenorhabditis elegans* [8–13]. MicroRNA (miRNA) was coined as the name for this new group of RNAs, and followed by diligent hunt for more, many other microRNAs were identified. Like miRNAs which were discovered first—lin-4 and let-7—many miRNAs were time- or site-specific, meaning they serve their function in some periods of life or only in some cell types [14, 15]. Targets of these RNAs were found in more than 60% of human protein-coding genes [16]. Together with their specific level necessary for fulfilling their job, it was inevitable to notice possible role of ncRNAs in the development of various diseases.

Of all ncRNAs known so far, miRNAs occupy exceptional position, considering the amount of knowledge on their role in pathogenesis of cancer; therefore, their biogenesis, function, and predictive potential will be discussed in the subsequent lines. Following will be lncRNAs, for their potential to be used as a biomarker has been studied extensively in recent years, even though their association with cancer has been outlined already in the very first publications on lncRNAs [5].

This chapter is therefore focused on the potential application of noncoding RNAs in prediction of therapeutic response to tyrosine kinase inhibitors commonly used as targeted therapy in a wide range of metastatic cancers.

2. Noncoding RNAs and their role in cancer

2.1 Classification

Noncoding RNAs (ncRNAs) are usually divided into two groups according to their length. The term small ncRNA (sncRNA) is reserved for diverse group of transcripts shorter than 200 nucleotides. Longer transcripts above 200 nucleotides of length are called long ncRNA (lncRNA). Both short and long ncRNAs usually do not possess any protein-coding capacity [17] which is the main difference from mRNA; there are, however, some cases of cryptic reading frames in longer ncRNAs [18] and even translation of short functional micropeptides from transcripts formerly annotated as noncoding [19].

In contrast to sncRNA, spectrum of lncRNAs is much broader in possible length and thus also in sequence, structure, and function; therefore, similarities with protein-coding mRNA are highly variable with many exceptions among numerous types of noncoding transcripts [20]. Classification of lncRNAs is now more than imperfect due to limited understanding of this group with many structural and functional families unknown yet [21].

For some types of ncRNA, known sequences and their annotations [22] are gathered in online databases. miRbase.org has been established in 2006 as a first noncoding RNA registry for microRNA [23] following the formation of a unified nomenclature for miRNA.

Catalog of lncRNAs has been created much later, in 2012, under the domain mitranscriptome.org and contains data acquired with high-throughput RNA sequencing [24], combining results from several published sources such as The Cancer Genome Atlas [25] or the GENCODE project [21, 24].

2.2 Biogenesis

2.2.1 microRNA

miRNAs are 19–24 nucleotides long endogenously produced regulatory RNAs. Canonical pathway starts with RNA polymerase II which typically transcribes miRNA sequences, creating capped and polyadenylated primary miRNAs (pri-miRNAs) several hundred nucleotides long. Future mature miRNA sequence resides in the stem region of the secondary hairpin structure of pri-miRNA.

In the next step, pri-miRNA is spliced by a microprocessor complex to one or several hairpins each containing one future mature miRNA sequence—precursor miRNA (pre-miRNA) with its characteristic 5′phosphate and overhang of two nucleotides at 3′OH end. The microprocessor complex comprises mainly of RNase III enzyme Drosha [26] and dimer of protein DiGeorge critical region 8 (DGCR8 or known as Pasha in flies) able to bind double-stranded RNA (dsRNA) [27, 28].

Pre-miRNA is further processed in the cytoplasm, and to get there, it is bound by nuclear transporter protein Exportin 5 [29] and transferred out of the nucleus. In the cytoplasm, pre-miRNA is cleaved by another RNAse III-type enzyme Dicer in cooperation with other proteins depending on species; in humans, for example, it is *trans*-activation-responsive RNA-binding protein (TRBP) [30]. Pre-miRNA is cleaved at stem sequence close to the terminal loop, creating double-stranded RNA intermediate. Depending on several factors such as thermodynamic stability, one of the strands is then recruited into an RNA-induced silencing complex (RISC) by binding with protein Argonaute (AGO) [30], such strand is termed leading. The other, which is thermodynamically more stable, called passenger strand, is usually discarded but can also act in complex with Ago as functional miRNA [31].

Canonical pathway, however, can be overcome, and miRNAs can be produced in alternative, noncanonical ways [32]. Alternative routes independent on various parts of the canonical biogenesis have been described before [33–35], and it is known that they give rise to some other types of sncRNA such as snoRNA or endogenous short hairpin RNAs (shRNAs).

2.2.2 Long noncoding RNA

Due to their highly variable structure and function, it is difficult to outline a general biogenesis pathway for lncRNA. At least part of the biogenesis is shared among lncRNAs and protein-coding mRNAs [21], including transcription by RNA polymerase II and chromatin modifications as those seen during transcription of protein-coding sequences, for example, methylation and acetylation of histones in active promoters [36]. The main differences lie in fewer but usually longer exons in lncRNAs [21], more tissue-specific expression [20], and abundance in the nucleus rather than the cytoplasm [36, 37].

Enormous variability of noncoding RNAs is achieved more on posttranscriptional level than by individual transcriptional mechanisms. Besides standard processes such as polyadenylation, capping, and splicing, nascent ncRNAs undergo modifications that are not typical for mRNAs. Cleaving of 3′end by RNAse P is a typical modification in the biogenesis of metastasis-associated lung adenocarcinoma transcript 1 (MALAT1) while creating short tRNA-like transcript (MATAL1-associated small cytoplasmic RNA—mascRNA) and mature lncRNA. Another variation of standard pre-mRNA splicing is the back-splicing of previously spliced transcript creating a circular lncRNA (circRNA). Spliced-out introns can also gain lncRNA status when they escape degradation and then function as lariat-shaped circular RNAs [38, 39]. After all, even miRNAs, as much as other sncRNAs, arise from primary long transcripts which are classifiable as lncRNA but are processed by following miRNA biogenesis pathway [39]. Evidence also suggests that transcriptional apparatus of miRNAs is somehow involved in expression of lncRNAs, too, as knockout of Dicer leads to downregulation of not only miRNAs but also lncRNAs as a class [40].

2.3 Cellular functions and roles in cancer

Distinct length of miRNA predestines them for a specific cellular function. The so-called seed region of miRNA sequence recognizes its target mRNA and binds complementary to its 3′untranslated region. miRNA-mRNA interaction leads to repression of the translation by destabilization of the target mRNA or by recruiting the mRNA degradation factors. As a result, expression of the target is decreased [41]. As the seed region of miRNA is only eight nucleotides long, recognized sequence will not be very specific—many different target mRNAs can contain identical eight-nucleotide combination. miRNAs are therefore pleiotropic in their effect, creating an intertwined posttranscriptional regulatory network. sncRNAs however expand their impact beyond posttranscriptional downregulation of expression. Other types of sncRNAs such as PiWi-interacting RNAs or siRNAs facilitate various cellular functions through pathway of RNA interference and its components. Transposon gene silencing, maturation of rRNA or histone pre-mRNA, and guiding of various complexes to a certain site are only some of very specific functions of short transcripts in cell [42].

In lncRNAs, the range of cellular roles is considerably wider, affecting processes spanning from transcription to epigenetic modification.

LncRNAs regulate transcription in *cis* (genes on the same chromosome) or *trans* (genes on another chromosome) manner acting through transcriptional interference, for example, by overlapping promoters or by binding to transcription factors [43, 44].

Of posttranscriptional modifications, lncRNAs are involved in pre-mRNA capping and polyadenylation, necessary for proper mRNA translation and mRNA splicing, the processes indispensable for diverse protein products from rather small choice of protein-coding sequences in higher eukaryotes [43]. lncRNAs are involved also in epigenetic regulation by loss of imprinting or changes in methylation patterns of cytosine residues in CpG dinucleotide islands. Chromatin remodeling is facilitated by lncRNA, too, as they can recruit chromatin-remodeling and histone-modifying enzymes [43, 45].

Like miRNA, lncRNA can affect mRNA half-life and its stability, consequently triggering mRNA decay or repression of translation by imperfect pairing; on the contrary, perfect pairing can protect the target mRNA from degradation. Moreover, lncRNAs can affect miRNA network by acting as miRNA decoys or cause forming of endogenous siRNAs [43, 46].

The processes stated above are just few of many cellular actions affected by ncRNAs. Mere expression of a gene, protein-coding or not, is only a first step in a working cellular environment which is achieved by fine tuning and multiple layers of control facilitated by ncRNAs on transcriptional and posttranscriptional level. Although different from their targets, ncRNAs suffer from the same errors and damages as protein-coding sequences. Deregulated levels of ncRNAs are mostly observed either because given ncRNA is a target of upstream mutated or epigenetically deregulated effector oncogene, as a result of mutation in ncRNA sequence or defects in transcription and posttranscriptional editing and splicing. Either way, disruption of this network can add to imbalances in critical nodes such as DNA damage repair, cell division, and response to mitogenic and proapoptotic signals, thus shifting cells to precancerous phenotypes.

The genome-wide studies to localize miRNA genes in human genome found that miRNAs are frequently localized at fragile sites, minimal regions of heterozygous loss or amplification, or common breakpoint regions in human cancer [45]. Besides the structural and genetic alterations, the epigenetic silencing of miRNAs genes by DNA promoter hypermethylation or histone hypoacetylation has been described in some solid tumors and hematologic malignancies. Whole-genome miRNA expression analysis clearly showed that the aberrant miRNA expression patterns present a common feature in the various tumor types. Based on these studies, deregulation of miRNAs was declared to be an important event in the initiation and progression of many cancers. Considering the network of targeted mRNAs and miRNA expression changes, miRNA can be classified as oncogenic miRNA or tumor-suppressive miRNA; some miRNAs may exhibit both features dependently on the cellular context in various cancers [45].

3. Noncoding RNAs as predictive biomarkers of therapeutic response

Drug resistance, either primary or developed secondary, is a crucial factor in tumor recurrence and poor outcome. Administration of the best of current therapies to a group of patients with similar symptoms and seemingly identical diagnosis has shown itself to be inefficient as there is almost always a subgroup of patients not benefiting from the treatment. With ever more precise options in molecular description of patients, it has become evident that cancer is not a single disease, but large family of heterogenous diseases asking for an individual approach. Even after onset of targeted therapy, incomparably more specific than conventional chemo- and radiotherapy, the problem of non-responding subgroups of patients remained. Histological classification was insufficient in prediction of what would be the most effective treatment for a given patient.

To be considered a feasible biomarker, a molecule needs to meet several criteria. Its expression must be cell-type- or tissue-specific and significantly altered during the disease or studied condition compared to normal state. Predictive biomarker then should provide an information on therapeutic outcome in a given patient before the treatment administration, and it could manifest itself in a form of up- and downregulations of RNA or protein expression level, gene copies, mutations, and signaling signatures either downstream or in parallel and can be derived retrospectively or prospectively [47]. For obvious reasons, before ncRNAs, various proteins in the blood and tissue, gene mutations, and later mRNA transcripts were prominent candidates as predictive biomarkers. Up to now, several genetic variants (e.g., SNPs in VEGF-A, VEGF-R1, VEGF-R3, and FGF-R2; [48]) were associated, for example, with response to sunitinib, pazopanib, sorafenib, or axitinib response. Histological and molecular features are also potential biomarkers, in addition to other such as protein expression and immune response activation (e.g., differential levels of some cytokines like IL-6 were observed in patients with progressive disease, although with insignificant results). Also, epigenetic factors such as methylation status were studied; for example, hypermethylation of cystatin-M gene (CST6) and leukocyte adhesion deficiency-1 (LAD1) were observed in patients with shorter PFS on TKI therapy (all reviewed in [48]). Although many molecules have been considered as biomarker candidates, only a few of them have really made it to clinical practice mostly due to lack of proper validation on significant cohorts and study design discrepancies. Also, in some cases, it is not clear whether given molecule has prognostic or rather predictive character.

With the discovery of miRNA and their regulatory impact, attention has been turned to ncRNAs. Concerning miRNAs, the first attempts in finding cancer-specific ncRNA biomarkers were made in Carlo Croce's research group in 2002 [49]. A team of researchers discovered that miR-15 and miR-16 sequences lie in a region frequently deleted in chronic lymphocytic leukemia (CLL) and this deletion leads to downregulation of these miRNAs. Further investigation revealed that many microRNA genes are located at fragile genomic regions and that microRNA profiles show specific patterns correlating with distinct clinical subtypes of CLL [50, 51]. In this case, microRNAs were the first ncRNAs tested for biomarker potential, but many more different kinds of noncoding RNAs emerged throughout the years, mostly after next-generation sequencing was introduced. Advances in high-throughput profiling technologies led to discovery of over 1900 mature human miRNAs from more than 1500 miRNA gene loci [23] and were followed by numerous studies focused on application of ncRNAs as diagnostic, prognostic, and predictive markers or therapeutic targets. To name just a few of many examples of promising biomarkers [52, 53], long intergenic RNA named HOX transcript antisense RNA (HOTAIR) is known to be metastasis-associated in breast cancer and playing active role in modulating cancer epigenome [54]. Choosing from sncRNAs, one example out of many could be miR-126 which has been shown to be involved in VEGF/PI3K/Akt/MRP1 signaling pathway as a principal player directly binding to vascular endothelial growth factor A (VEGF-A) [55]. Another one is miR-31, a potent factor in the development of various tumors with many target genes [56] which has been shown in many studies to be a reliable biomarker of response to anti-EGFR therapy. Recent large randomized trials proved low expression of miR-31 is an indicator of longer response and overall survival of patients with advanced colorectal carcinoma and wild-type allele of KRAS [57–59]. As for therapeutical applications, phase I study of MRX34, a liposomal miR-34a mimic, has been finished in 2017 with promising results in treatment of various solid tumors [60].

Reasons for extensive biomarker research on ncRNAs are their unique attributes beating proteins and mRNAs as biomarkers. In comparison, ncRNAs often manifest higher tissue-specific expression patterns which are necessary for precise distinction between different molecular subtypes of the disease and avoiding false-positive or false-negative results. Among the important characteristics of promising biomarkers is their detection in samples obtained noninvasively. Overall trend is to get as many and as detailed information with minimal burden for patients. Although ncRNAs are easily detectable in tissue samples (either fresh frozen or formalin-fixed paraffin-embedded), they are released and circulating in body fluids such as the blood, plasma, saliva, or urine as well which is incomparably less painful and faster to obtain than tissue specimens. This would be of tremendous value, for example, for patients with lung cancer who are routinely recommended for molecular testing for mutational status of epidermal growth factor receptor (EGFR) and anaplastic lymphoma receptor tyrosine kinase (ALK) in order to identify patients with superior response to TKIs so that they can avoid conventional chemotherapy. However, to obtain accurate lung biopsies for such testing, patients experience severe discomfort during difficult invasive procedures. Liquid biopsies would be thus much convenient option [61].

Replicative nature of ncRNAs makes them easy to detect by polymerase chain reaction and various modifications of this method, also microarrays and sequencing. ncRNAs vary in stability according to their length, secondary structure, association with proteins, or protection by exosomes; however, there is a consensus that relative to DNA or mRNA, shorter ncRNAs are more stable and less likely to be cleaved by RNAses or to be degraded by environmental agents such as storing temperature [62]. There are however some limits and variability between different types of sample handling and storage [63].

Based on many functions and pleiotropic character of ncRNAs, their involvement in progression of cancer and in modulation of therapeutic response is not surprising. In the following lines, we provide an overview (**Table 1**) of ncRNAs currently known to play a role in the development of resistance to TKIs, and what is more, their level seems to be an indicator of such resistance.

Drug	ncRNA	Deregulation in drug-resistant patients	Diagnosis	Technological platform	Study
Sunitinib	miR-1307-3p + miR-425-5p	Up	RCC (all)	NGS, qPCR	García-Donas et al. [64]
	miR-942 + miR-133 model	Up		qPCR	Kovacova et al. [65]
	miR-942	Up		qPCR array	Prior et al. [66]
	miR-628-5p miR-23b miR-27b	Down		qPCR	Puente et al. [67]
	miR-99-5p	Down		NGS, qPCR	Lukamowicz-Rajska et al. [68]
	miR-9-5p	Up		TaqMan-MicroRNA Cards, qPcr, digital PCR	Ralla et al. [69]
	miR-141	Down		qPCR array	Berkers et al. [70]
	miR-424c	Down		Microarray, qPCR	Gámez-Pozo et al. [71]
	miR-1 + miR-597 model	Up		qPCR array	Khella et al. [72]
	miR-155 miR-484	Up		qPCR array	Merhautova et al. [73]
Sorafenib	SRLR	Up	RCC	Microarray, qPCR	Xu et al. [84]
	miR-425-3p	Down	HCC	TaqMan low density array, qPCR	Vaira et al. [83]
Gefitinib	miR-21	Up	NSCLC	Microarray qPCR	Shen et al. [74]
	EGFR-AS1	Up	HNSC	qPCR, NanoString panel	Tan et al. [85]
	miR-630	Down	LUAD	qPCR	Wu et al. [88]
	miR-200c	Down	NSCLC	qPCR	Li et al. [75]
	MiG6-miR-200 ratio	Up	NSCLC, BC	qPCR	Izumchenko et al. [76]
Erlotinib	miR-630	Down	LUAD	qPCR	Wu et al. [77]
	miR-223	Up	NSCLC	Microarray, FirePlex	Joerger et al. [78]
	miR-200c	Down	NSCLC	qPCR	Li et al. [75]
	EGFR-AS1	Up	HNSC	qPCR, NanoString panel	Tan et al. [85]
	MiG6-miR-200 ratio	Up	NSCLC, BC	qPCR	Izumchenko et al. [76]

Drug	ncRNA	Deregulation in drug-resistant patients	Diagnosis	Technological platform	Study
Lapatinib	miR-16	Down	BRCA, STAD	Microarray, qPCR	Venturutti et al. [86]
	miR-630	Down	BRCA	qPCRC	Corcoran et al. [79]
Nintedanib	miR-200 family	Down	LUAD	qPCR array	Nishijima et al. [80]
Neratinib	miR-630	Down	BRCA	qPCRC	Corcoran et al. [79]
Afatinib	miR-630	Down	BRCA	qPCRC	Corcoran et al. [79]

mRCC, metastatic renal cell carcinoma; RCC, renal cell carcinoma; HCC, hepatocellular carcinoma; NSCLC, non-small cell lung carcinoma; HNSC, head and neck squamous carcinoma; LUAD, lung adenocarcinoma; BRCA, breast invasive carcinoma; BC, breast carcinoma; STAD, stomach adenocarcinoma.

Table 1.
Overview of potential ncRNA biomarkers of response to tyrosine kinase inhibitors.

3.1 Sunitinib

Most studies on prediction of response by miRNA levels have been carried out on renal cell carcinoma and sunitinib as a prominent treatment choice in patients with clear cell renal cell carcinoma. Ten papers have been published so far on prediction of sunitinib response in metastatic renal cell carcinoma (mRCC). Though there are some discrepancies in experimental design, mainly in samples and technologies used in explorative phase, most of the studies are carried out on a rather small cohort; there is some overlap in results. miR-484, miR-221/222, miR-942, miR-133a, miR-628-5p, and miR-155-5p were successfully validated by more than one study; however, none of them turned out to be significantly deregulated in all the studies [64–73].

It is useful to have some information about mechanistic impact of predictive miRNAs, because usually their deregulation is somehow connected with the development of therapy resistance. For example, in the work of Puente et al., two of three significantly deregulated miRNAs, miR-23b and miR-27b, are known to inhibit Notch1 and c-Met pointing on potential involvement of Notch pathway in sunitinib response, serving as solid base for future research. In some cases, however, the targets of predictive miRNAs are waiting to be characterized and subjected to a further functional analysis of mechanistic connection of a given miRNA with response to sunitinib. In other work [77], miR-99b-5p has been discovered to be significantly lower in patients with shorter progression-free survival; unfortunately they did not manage to validate it in an independent cohort by RT-qPCR with sufficient statistical significance. However, miRNAs from miR-99 family are possibly tumor suppressors not only in RCC; there is evidence of their involvement in OSCC in regulation of IGF1R [81].

3.2 Sorafenib

Primarily used for treatment of RCC, sorafenib is ineffective in patients with initial resistance, which can be predicted by expression levels of sorafenib resistance-associated lncRNA (SRLR) identified by Xu et al. [82]. lncRNA-SRLR level has been correlated with sorafenib therapy response in RCC patients, and clear connection has been demonstrated. Manipulation with its expression leads to changes in response of RCC cell lines. According to recent findings, SRLR acts through IL-6/STAT3 pathway and by binding to NF-κB promotes IL-6 transcription and activation of STAT3, in the end causing the development of sorafenib resistance [82]. To prove that, researchers introduced STAT3 inhibitor and IL-6-receptor antagonist, which restored response to the treatment.

In another study on patients with hepatocellular carcinoma [83], six miRNAs have been significantly associated with progression-free survival (PFS); however, only miR-425-3p was successfully validated. Higher levels of this miRNA indicated longer PFS. In vitro tests have shown reduced cell motility and increased cell death in HCC cell lines when miR-425-3p was added which indicates that miR-425-3p probably acts as tumor suppressor [83].

3.2.1 Gefitinib, erlotinib, and nintedanib

There are known some mutations in epidermal growth factor receptor (EGFR) which are reliable indicator of response to EGFR-targeting TKIs. However, these mutations are minor, and for patients with wild-type EGFR, there is no biomarker of response to the treatment [84].

Quite robust has been a study of non-small cellular lung carcinoma (NSCLC) patients treated with gefitinib [74], where miR-21 has been proven to be a potent biomarker of response. The study has been carried out on 128 radically resected patients in explorative phase compared to 32 healthy controls; results have been validated on 201 EGFR-mutated patients. In patients with better therapy outcome, miR-21 has been significantly reduced.

Tan et al. [85] showed interesting case report of two patients with exceptional response to gefitinib, diagnosed with head and neck squamous cell carcinoma. Silent mutation in lncRNA epidermal growth factor receptor—associated 1 (EGFR-AS1)—led to destabilization of this lncRNA which in turn shifted splicing of EGFR to isoform D and noncanonical EGFR addiction, thus affecting its sensitivity to tyrosine kinase inhibitors.

Gefitinib and erlotinib are frequently used in EGFR-mutated lung adenocarcinoma where they reach better results and longer progression-free survival than in wild-type-EGFR lung adenocarcinoma patients. However, in both cases the development of resistance to treatment is inevitable; still its mechanism remains uncovered. The first information on the development of resistance was shown by Wu et al. [77]. miR-630 and one of its target transcripts, YAP1, create a feedback loop with ERK and are suspected to be responsible for the resistance in EGFR-mutated adenocarcinoma cells. Further they showed that low level of miR-630 indicates future resistance to TKIs in EGFR-mutated patients with lung adenocarcinoma.

Erlotinib alone has been studied in phase II clinical trial of Swiss Group for Clinical Cancer Research (SAKK) on blood samples of NSCLC patients treated with first-line combination of bevacizumab and erlotinib followed by chemotherapy. The study was focused on circulating miRNAs, and their main objective was to find prognostic miRNAs, but they identified also some predictive miRNAs both for targeted therapy and chemotherapy. miR-223 expression was shown to have the highest predictive value for disease stabilization and time to progression, with higher expression being associated with worse outcome [78].

Among other miRNAs, miR-200 family seems to have extensive impact on response to nintedanib, gefitinib, and erlotinib. Nintedanib is a multi-targeted angiokinase inhibitor prescribed for idiopathic pulmonary fibrosis and advanced

NSCLC [80]. It has been shown in work on lung cancer cell lines (5 nintedanib-resistant/5 nintedanib-sensitive) that some miRNAs belonging to miR-200 family (miR-200, miR-200a, and miR-141) are significantly lower in nintedanib-resistant cells. Induction of miR-200 and miR-141 has led to restored treatment sensitivity in resistant cells. miR-200/ZEB axis might play a role in resistance to treatment and serves as a potential biomarker of response to nintedanib. The work also proved some role of this family in EMT transition which has been outlined before in Izumchenko et al. [76] where miR-200 has been suggested to play a role in TGFβ-miR200-MIG6 axis. According to their findings, authors concluded that this pathway creates an EMT-associated switch-inducing resistance to EGFR-targeting drugs. Further, they observed that the ratio of MIG6 versus miR-200 expression indicates response to erlotinib.

Yet another work connected miR-200c with response to erlotinib and gefitinib in patients with NSCLC. When upregulated, miR-200c correlates with sensitivity to gefitinib in EGFR wild-type cell lines. Besides other pathways leading to EMT, in this work it has been shown that miR-200c regulates EMT also through PI3K/AKT pathway and MEK/WRK. One hundred fifty patients treated with gefitinib or erlotinib as a second- or third-line treatment were tested in this study, and in 66 NSCLC patients with wild-type EGFR, high levels of miR-200c expression were associated with higher disease control rate (DCR), longer progression-free survival (PFS), and longer overall survival (OS) than low miR-200c expression subgroup [75].

3.2.2 Lapatinib

MiR-16 mediates trastuzumab and lapatinib response, as shown on trastuzumab- and lapatinib-resistant breast and gastric cancer cell cultures [86]. Artificial increase of miR-16 expression had an inhibitory effect on cell growth in vitro, and it is speculated that expression of miR-16 is regulated by phosphatidylinositol 3 kinase (PI3K)/AKT pathway starting at extracellular signal regulated kinases 1/2 (ERK1/2) which are blocked by trastuzumab and lapatinib. Probably due to inhibition of c-Myc which is downregulated by PI3K/AKT, the level of miR-16 is then upregulated to normal level and inhibits proliferation of both breast cancer and gastric cancer cells. The same effect was achieved by artificial increase of miR-16, as stated above, indicating that miR-16 is not only a biomarker but possible therapeutic target, too.

3.2.3 HER-targeting drugs

miR-630, as mentioned above, has been linked also to response to HER-targeting drugs, namely, lapatinib, neratinib, and afatinib, used in breast and lung cancer. The same problem as elsewhere repeats itself also in these diagnosis—targeting of HER in HER2 overexpressing patients is mostly effective, except in patients with primary or secondary resistance. Response to these drugs is mediated by IGF1R which is targeted by miR-630. Work of Corcoran et al. [79] shows that an artificial increase of miR-630 in cells with primary or secondary resistance to anti-HER therapy leads to restored efficacy of such drugs. Blocking of miR-630 leads to the development of resistance. Results were validated also on set of tumor and non-tumor tissue. According to current knowledge, miR-630 plays a dual role in apoptosis and drug resistance, because depending on cell type, it serves as a tumor suppressor in breast carcinoma [87] and hepatocellular carcinoma [88] or as an oncogene in renal cell carcinoma [89].

4. Conclusions

Noncoding RNAs gained extensive attention in recent years for their unique features as endogenous regulators of gene expression, potential biomarkers, and therapeutic targets. Tissue specificity, stability, and detectability in all types of tissues and body fluids predestine them to become very promising biomarkers applicable in personalized medicine. Major attention has been devoted to miRNAs; less is known about involvement of lncRNAs. Although studies on profiling and feasibility of various ncRNAs as diagnostic, prognostic, and predictive biomarkers are accumulating, none have made it to real clinical practice so far. Here we provide an overview of current knowledge on possible biomarkers of response to tyrosine kinase inhibitors, a breakthrough targeted therapy of several solid tumors. Currently, besides studies focused on sunitinib, there are rather solitary results acquired on small cohorts of less than 100 patients; therefore, it is difficult to come up with any conclusions. Even if there are more studies on response prediction of one therapeutic agent, inter-study discrepancies in validated biomarkers are significant, and results overlap sparsely. This can be ascribed to differences in study design such as type of samples, technology, normalization, statistical analysis, thresholds, and cutoff values set as criteria for stratification of patients and many more. Out of all TKI, sunitinib is much more ahead in terms of number of biomarker studies, study design similarity, and partial overlap of the results.

In spite all of that, miR-200 family, miR-221/222, miR-484, miR-221/222, miR-942, miR-133a, miR-628-5p, miR-155-5p, and miR-630 seem to have significant biomarker potential indicated by several studies. However, independent prospective validation on larger cohorts taking utmost account of study design in previous relevant studies is necessary for future clinical application of miRNA-based biomarker technology to TKIs' therapeutic response prediction.

Acknowledgements

This publication was supported by the Ministry of Health of the Czech Republic, grant no. 15-34678A.

Conflict of interest

The authors whose names are listed immediately below certify that they have no affiliations with or involvement in any organization or entity with any financial interest (such as honoraria; educational grants; participation in speakers' bureaus; membership, employment, consultancies, stock ownership, or other equity interest; and expert testimony or patent-licensing arrangements) or nonfinancial interest (such as personal or professional relationships, affiliations, knowledge, or beliefs) in the subject matter or materials discussed in this manuscript.

Author details

Julia Kovacova and Ondrej Slaby*
Central European Institute of Technology, Masaryk University, Brno, Czech Republic

*Address all correspondence to: on.slaby@gmail.com

References

[1] Wise JA, Weiner AM. Dictyostelium small nuclear RNA D2 is homologous to rat nucleolar RNA U3 and is encoded by a dispersed multigene family. Cell. 1980;**22**(1 Pt 1):109-118

[2] Calvet JP, Pederson T. Base-pairing interactions between small nuclear RNAs and nuclear RNA precursors as revealed by psoralen cross-linking in vivo. Cell. 1981;**26**(3 Pt 1):363-370

[3] Calvet JP, Meyer LM, Pederson T. Small nuclear RNA U2 is base-paired to heterogeneous nuclear RNA. Science. 1982;**217**(4558):456-458

[4] Lacoste-Royal G, Simard R. Localization of small nuclear RNA by EM autoradiography in Chinese hamster ovary (CHO) cells. Experimental Cell Research. 1983;**149**(2):311-323

[5] Elkin M, Shevelev A, Schulze E, Tykocinsky M, Cooper M, Ariel I, et al. The expression of the imprinted H19 and IGF-2 genes in human bladder carcinoma. FEBS Letters. 1995;**374**(1):57-61

[6] Smith CM, Steitz JA. Classification of gas5 as a multi-small-nucleolar-RNA (snoRNA) host gene and a member of the 5'-terminal oligopyrimidine gene family reveals common features of snoRNA host genes. Molecular and Cellular Biology. 1998;**18**(12):6897-6909

[7] Bussemakers MJ, van Bokhoven A, Verhaegh GW, Smit FP, Karthaus HF, Schalken JA, et al. DD3: A new prostate-specific gene, highly overexpressed in prostate cancer. Cancer Research. 1999;**59**(23):5975-5979

[8] Brannan CI, Dees EC, Ingram RS, Tilghman SM. The product of the H19 gene may function as an RNA. Molecular and Cellular Biology. 1990;**10**(1):28-36

[9] Brown CJ, Ballabio A, Rupert JL, Lafreniere RG, Grompe M, Tonlorenzi R, et al. A gene from the region of the human X inactivation centre is expressed exclusively from the inactive X chromosome. Nature. 1991;**349**(6304):38-44

[10] Fire A, Albertson D, Harrison SW, Moerman DG. Production of antisense RNA leads to effective and specific inhibition of gene expression in *C. elegans* muscle. Development. 1991;**113**(2):503-514

[11] Fire A, Xu S, Montgomery MK, Kostas SA, Driver SE, Mello CC. Potent and specific genetic interference by double-stranded RNA in *Caenorhabditis elegans*. Nature. 1998;**391**(6669):806-811

[12] Lee RC, Feinbaum RL, Ambros V. The *C. elegans* heterochronic gene lin-4 encodes small RNAs with antisense complementarity to lin-14. Cell. 1993;**75**(5):843-854

[13] Reinhart BJ, Slack FJ, Basson M, Pasquinelli AE, Bettinger JC, Rougvie AE, et al. The 21-nucleotide let-7 RNA regulates developmental timing in *Caenorhabditis elegans*. Nature. 2000;**403**(6772):901-906

[14] Slack FJ, Basson M, Liu Z, Ambros V, Horvitz HR, Ruvkun G. The lin-41 RBCC gene acts in the *C. elegans* heterochronic pathway between the let-7 regulatory RNA and the LIN-29 transcription factor. Molecular Cell. 2000;**5**(4):659-669

[15] Pasquinelli AE, Reinhart BJ, Slack F, Martindale MQ, Kuroda MI, Maller B, et al. Conservation of the sequence and temporal expression of let-7 heterochronic regulatory RNA. Nature. 2000;**408**(6808):86-89

[16] Friedman RC, Farh KKH, Burge CB, Bartel DP. Most mammalian mRNAs

are conserved targets of microRNAs. Genome Research. 2009;**19**(1):92-105

[17] Jia H, Osak M, Bogu GK, Stanton LW, Johnson R, Lipovich L. Genome-wide computational identification and manual annotation of human long noncoding RNA genes. RNA. 2010;**16**(8):1478-1487

[18] Bánfai B, Jia H, Khatun J, Wood E, Risk B, Gundling WE, et al. Long noncoding RNAs are rarely translated in two human cell lines. Genome Research. 2012;**22**(9):1646-1657

[19] Anderson DM, Anderson KM, Chang CL, Makarewich CA, Nelson BR, McAnally JR, et al. A micropeptide encoded by a putative long noncoding RNA regulates muscle performance. Cell. 2015;**160**(4):595-606

[20] Cabili MN, Trapnell C, Goff L, Koziol M, Tazon-Vega B, Regev A, et al. Integrative annotation of human large intergenic noncoding RNAs reveals global properties and specific subclasses. Genes and Development. 2011;**25**(18):1915-1927

[21] Derrien T, Johnson R, Bussotti G, Tanzer A, Djebali S, Tilgner H, et al. The GENCODE v7 catalog of human long noncoding RNAs: Analysis of their gene structure, evolution, and expression. Genome Research. 2012;**22**(9):1775-1789

[22] Ambros V, Bartel B, Bartel DP, Burge CB, Carrington JC, Chen X, et al. A uniform system for microRNA annotation. RNA. 2003;**9**(3):277-279

[23] Kozomara A, Griffiths-Jones S. miRBase: Annotating high confidence microRNAs using deep sequencing data. Nucleic Acids Research. 2014;**42**(D1):D68-D73

[24] Harrow J, Frankish A, Gonzalez JM, Tapanari E, Diekhans M, Kokocinski F, et al. GENCODE: The reference human genome annotation for the ENCODE project. Genome Research. 2012;**22**(9):1760-1774

[25] Cancer Genome Atlas Research Network, Weinstein JN, Collisson EA, Mills GB, Shaw KRM, Ozenberger BA, et al. The cancer genome Atlas Pan-Cancer analysis project. Nature Genetics. 2013;**45**(10):1113-1120

[26] Lee Y, Ahn C, Han J, Choi H, Kim J, Yim J, et al. The nuclear RNase III drosha initiates microRNA processing. Nature. 2003;**425**(6956):415-419

[27] Han J, Lee Y, Yeom KH, Kim YK, Jin H, Kim VN. The drosha-DGCR8 complex in primary microRNA processing. Genes and Development. 2004;**18**(24):3016-3027

[28] Landthaler M, Yalcin A, Tuschl T. The human diGeorge syndrome critical region gene 8 and its *D. melanogaster* homolog are required for miRNA biogenesis. Current Biology. 2004;**14**(23):2162-2167

[29] Yi R, Qin Y, Macara IG, Cullen BR. Exportin-5 mediates the nuclear export of pre-microRNAs and short hairpin RNAs. Genes and Develpoment. 2003;**17**(24):3011-3016

[30] Chendrimada TP, Gregory RI, Kumaraswamy E, Norman J, Cooch N, Nishikura K, et al. TRBP recruits the dicer complex to Ago2 for microRNA processing and gene silencing. Nature. 2005;**436**(7051):740-744

[31] Okamura K, Liu N, Lai EC. Distinct mechanisms for microRNA strand selection by *Drosophila argonautes*. Molecular Cell. 2009;**36**(3):431-444

[32] Kim YK, Kim B, Kim VN. Re-evaluation of the roles of DROSHA, Export in 5, and DICER in microRNA biogenesis. Proceedings of the National Academy of Sciences of the United States of America. 2016;**113**(13):E1881-E1889

[33] Babiarz JE, Ruby JG, Wang Y, Bartel DP, Blelloch R, Mouse ES. Cells express endogenous shRNAs, siRNAs, and other microprocessor-independent, dicer-dependent small RNAs. Genes and Development. 2008;**22**(20):2773-2785

[34] Ender C, Krek A, Friedländer MR, Beitzinger M, Weinmann L, Chen W, et al. A human snoRNA with microRNA-like functions. Molecular Cell. 2008;**32**(4):519-528

[35] Okamura K, Hagen JW, Duan H, Tyler DM, Lai EC. The mirtron pathway generates microRNA-class regulatory RNAs in drosophila. Cell. 2007;**130**(1):89-100

[36] Melé M, Mattioli K, Mallard W, Shechner DM, Gerhardinger C, Rinn JL. Chromatin environment, transcriptional regulation, and splicing distinguish lincRNAs and mRNAs. Genome Research. 2017;**27**(1):27-37

[37] Djebali S, Davis CA, Merkel A, Dobin A, Lassmann T, Mortazavi A, et al. Landscape of transcription in human cells. Nature. 2012;**489**(7414):101-108

[38] Quinn JJ, Chang HY. Unique features of long non-coding RNA biogenesis and function. Nature Reviews. Genetics. 2016;**17**(1):47-62

[39] Ulitsky I. Interactions between short and long noncoding RNAs. FEBS Letters. 2018;**592**(17):2874-2883

[40] Zheng GXY, Do BT, Webster DE, Khavari PA, Chang HY. Dicer-microRNA-Myc circuit promotes transcription of hundreds of long noncoding RNAs. Nature Structural and Molecular Biology. 2014;**21**(7):585-590

[41] MacFarlane L-A, Murphy PR. MicroRNA: Biogenesis, function and role in cancer. Current Genomics. 2010;**11**(7):537-561

[42] Martens-Uzunova ES, Olvedy M, Jenster G. Beyond microRNA – Novel RNAs derived from small non-coding RNA and their implication in cancer. Cancer Letters. 2013;**340**(2):201-211

[43] Kunej T, Obsteter J, Pogacar Z, Horvat S, Calin GA. The decalog of long non-coding RNA involvement in cancer diagnosis and monitoring. Critical Reviews in Clinical Laboratory Sciences. 2014;**51**(6):344-357

[44] Wang KC, Yang YW, Liu B, Sanyal A, Corces-Zimmerman R, Chen Y, et al. A long noncoding RNA maintains active chromatin to coordinate homeotic gene expression. Nature. 2011;**472**(7341):120-124

[45] Slaby O, Laga R, Sedlacek O. Therapeutic targeting of non-coding RNAs in cancer. The Biochemical Journal. 2017;**474**(24):4219-4251

[46] Watanabe T, Totoki Y, Toyoda A, Kaneda M, Kuramochi-Miyagawa S, Obata Y, et al. Endogenous siRNAs from naturally formed dsRNAs regulate transcripts in mouse oocytes. Nature. 2008;**453**(7194):539-543

[47] Lowery A, Han Z. Assessment of tumor response to tyrosine kinase inhibitors. Frontiers in Bioscience (Landmark Edition). 2011;**16**:1996-2007

[48] Diekstra MHM, Swen JJ, Gelderblom H, Guchelaar HJ. A decade of pharmacogenomics research on tyrosine kinase inhibitors in metastatic renal cell cancer: A systematic review. Expert Review of Molecular Diagnostics. 2016;**16**(5):605-618

[49] Calin GA, Dumitru CD, Shimizu M, Bichi R, Zupo S, Noch E, et al. Frequent deletions and down-regulation of micro-RNA genes miR15 and miR16 at 13q14 in chronic lymphocytic leukemia. Proceedings of the National Academy of Sciences of the United States of America. 2002;**99**(24):15524-15529

[50] Calin GA, Sevignani C, Dumitru CD, Hyslop T, Noch E, Yendamuri S, et al. Human microRNA genes are frequently located at fragile sites and genomic regions involved in cancers. Proceedings of the National Academy of Sciences of the United States of America. 2004;**101**(9):2999-3004

[51] Calin GA, Liu CG, Sevignani C, Ferracin M, Felli N, Dumitru CD, et al. MicroRNA profiling reveals distinct signatures in B cell chronic lymphocytic leukemias. Proceedings of the National Academy of Sciences of the United States of America. 2004;**101**(32):11755-11760

[52] Gutschner T, Richtig G, Haemmerle M, Pichler M. From biomarkers to therapeutic targets—the promises and perils of long non-coding RNAs in cancer. Cancer Metastasis Reviews. 2018;**37**(1):83-105

[53] Di Leva G, Garofalo M, Croce CM. MicroRNAs in cancer. Annual Review of Pathology. 2014;**9**:287-314

[54] Gupta RA, Shah N, Wang KC, Kim J, Horlings HM, Wong DJ, et al. Long non-coding RNA HOTAIR reprograms chromatin state to promote cancer metastasis. Nature. 2010;**464**(7291):1071-1076

[55] Zhu X, Li H, Long L, Hui L, Chen H, Wang X, et al. miR-126 enhances the sensitivity of non-small cell lung cancer cells to anticancer agents by targeting vascular endothelial growth factor A. Acta Biochimica et Biophysica Sinica. 2012;**44**(6):519-526

[56] Gao W, Liu L, Xu J, Shao Q, Liu Y, Zeng H, et al. A systematic analysis of predicted MiR-31-targets identifies a diagnostic and prognostic signature for lung cancer. Biomedicine and Pharmacotherapy. 2014;**68**(4):419-427

[57] Laurent-Puig P, Paget-Bailly S, Vernerey D, Vazart C, Decaulne V, Fontaine K, et al. Evaluation of miR 31 3p as a biomarker of prognosis and panitumumab benefit in RAS-wt advanced colorectal cancer (aCRC): Analysis of patients (pts) from the PICCOLO trial. Journal of Clinical Oncology. 2015;**33**(15_suppl):3547-3547

[58] Laurent-Puig P, Grisoni ML, Heinemann V, Bonnetain F, Fontaine K, Vazart C, et al. MiR 31 3p as a predictive biomarker of cetuximab efficacy effect in metastatic colorectal cancer (mCRC) patients enrolled in FIRE-3 study. Journal of Clinical Oncology. 2016;**34**(15_suppl):3516

[59] Laurent-Puig P, Grisoni ML, Heinemann V, Liebaert F, Neureiter D, Jung A, et al. Validation of miR-31-3p expression to predict Cetuximab efficacy when used as first-line treatment in RAS wild-type metastatic colorectal cancer. Clinical Cancer Research. 2018;clincanres.1324.2018. 2019;**25**(1):134-141. DOI: 10.1158/1078-0432.CCR-18-1324

[60] Beg MS, Brenner AJ, Sachdev J, Borad M, Kang YK, Stoudemire J, et al. Phase I study of MRX34, a liposomal miR-34a mimic, administered twice weekly in patients with advanced solid tumors. Investigational New Drugs. 2017;**35**(2):180-188

[61] Bernicker EH, Miller RA, Cagle PT. Biomarkers for selection of therapy for adenocarcinoma of the lung. Journal of Oncology Practice. 2017;**13**(4):221-227

[62] Balzano F, Deiana M, Dei Giudici S, Oggiano A, Baralla A, Pasella S, et al. miRNA stability in frozen plasma samples. Molecules. 2015;**20**(10):19030-19040

[63] Glinge C, Clauss S, Boddum K, Jabbari R, Jabbari J, Risgaard B, et al. Stability of circulating blood-based microRNAs - pre-analytic

methodological considerations. PLoS One. 2017;**12**(2):e0167969

[64] García-Donas J, Beuselinck B, Inglada-Pérez L, Graña O, Schöffski P, Wozniak A, et al. Deep sequencing reveals microRNAs predictive of antiangiogenic drug response. JCI Insight. 2016;**1**(10):e86051

[65] Kovacova J, Juracek J, Poprach A, Buchler T, Kopecky J, Fiala O, et al. Candidate microRNA biomarkers of therapeutic response to sunitinib in metastatic renal cell carcinoma: A validation study in patients with extremely good and poor response. Anticancer Research. 2018;**38**(5):2961-2965

[66] Prior C, Perez-Gracia JL, Garcia-Donas J, Rodriguez-Antona C, Guruceaga E, Esteban E, et al. Identification of tissue microRNAs predictive of sunitinib activity in patients with metastatic renal cell carcinoma. PLoS One. 2014;**9**(1):e86263

[67] Puente J, Laínez N, Dueñas M, Méndez-Vidal MJ, Esteban E, Castellano D, et al. Novel potential predictive markers of sunitinib outcomes in long-term responders versus primary refractory patients with metastatic clear-cell renal cell carcinoma. Oncotarget. 2017;**8**(18):30410-30421

[68] Lukamowicz-Rajska M, Mittmann C, Prummer M, Zhong Q, Bedke J, Hennenlotter J, et al. MiR-99b-5p expression and response to tyrosine kinase inhibitor treatment in clear cell renal cell carcinoma patients. Oncotarget. 2016;**7**(48):78433-78447

[69] Ralla B, Busch J, Flörcken A, Westermann J, Zhao Z, Kilic E, et al. miR-9-5p in nephrectomy specimens is a potential predictor of primary resistance to first-line treatment with tyrosine kinase inhibitors in patients with metastatic renal cell carcinoma. Cancers (Basel). 2018;**10**(9):pii: E321. DOI: 10.3390/cancers10090321

[70] Berkers J, Govaere O, Wolter P, Beuselinck B, Schöffski P, van Kempen LC, et al. A possible role for microRNA-141 down-regulation in sunitinib resistant metastatic clear cell renal cell carcinoma through induction of epithelial-to-mesenchymal transition and hypoxia resistance. Journal of Urology. 2013;**189**(5):1930-1938

[71] Gámez-Pozo A, Antón-Aparicio LM, Bayona C, Borrega P, Gallegos Sancho MI, García-Domínguez R, et al. MicroRNA expression profiling of peripheral blood samples predicts resistance to first-line sunitinib in advanced renal cell carcinoma patients. Neoplasia. 2012;**14**(12):1144-1152

[72] Khella HWZ, Butz H, Ding Q, Rotondo F, Evans KR, Kupchak P, et al. miR-221/222 are involved in response to sunitinib treatment in metastatic renal cell carcinoma. Molecular Therapy. 2015;**23**(11):1748-1758

[73] Merhautova J, Hezova R, Poprach A, Kovarikova A, Radova L, Svoboda M, et al. miR-155 and miR-484 are associated with time to progression in metastatic renal cell carcinoma treated with sunitinib. BioMed Research International. 2015;**2015**:941980

[74] Shen Y, Tang D, Yao R, Wang M, Wang Y, Yao Y, et al. microRNA expression profiles associated with survival, disease progression, and response to gefitinib in completely resected non-small-cell lung cancer with EGFR mutation. Medical Oncology. 2013;**30**(4):750

[75] Li J, Li X, Ren S, Chen X, Zhang Y, Zhou F, et al. miR-200c overexpression is associated with better efficacy of EGFR-TKIs in non-small cell lung cancer patients with EGFR wild-type. Oncotarget. 2014;**5**(17):7902-7916

[76] Izumchenko E, Chang X, Michailidi C, Kagohara L, Ravi R, Paz K, et al. The TGFβ-miR200-MIG6 pathway

orchestrates the EMT-associated kinase switch that induces resistance to EGFR inhibitors. Cancer Research. 2014;**74**(14):3995-4005

[77] Wu DW, Wang YC, Wang L, Chen CY, Lee H. A low microRNA-630 expression confers resistance to tyrosine kinase inhibitors in EGFR-mutated lung adenocarcinomas via miR-630/YAP1/ERK feedback loop. Theranostics. 2018;**8**(5):1256-1269

[78] Joerger M, Baty F, Früh M, Droege C, Stahel RA, Betticher DC, et al. Circulating microRNA profiling in patients with advanced non-squamous NSCLC receiving bevacizumab/erlotinib followed by platinum-based chemotherapy at progression (SAKK 19/05). Lung Cancer. 2014;**85**(2):306-313

[79] Corcoran C, Rani S, Breslin S, Gogarty M, Ghobrial IM, Crown J, et al. miR-630 targets IGF1R to regulate response to HER-targeting drugs and overall cancer cell progression in HER2 over-expressing breast cancer. Molecular Cancer. 2014;**13**:71

[80] Nishijima N, Seike M, Soeno C, Chiba M, Miyanaga A, Noro R, et al. miR-200/ZEB axis regulates sensitivity to nintedanib in non-small cell lung cancer cells. International Journal of Oncology. 2016;**48**(3):937-944

[81] Yen YC, Shiah SG, Chu HC, Hsu YM, Hsiao JR, Chang JY, et al. Reciprocal regulation of microRNA-99a and insulin-like growth factor I receptor signaling in oral squamous cell carcinoma cells. Molecular Cancer. 2014;**13**:6

[82] Xu Z, Yang F, Wei D, Liu B, Chen C, Bao Y, et al. Long noncoding RNA-SRLR elicits intrinsic sorafenib resistance via evoking IL-6/STAT3 axis in renal cell carcinoma. Oncogene. 2017;**36**(14):1965-1977

[83] Vaira V, Roncalli M, Carnaghi C, Faversani A, Maggioni M, Augello C, et al. MicroRNA-425-3p predicts response to sorafenib therapy in patients with hepatocellular carcinoma. Liver International. 2015;**35**(3):1077-1086

[84] Li X, Cai W, Yang G, Su C, Ren S, Zhao C, et al. Comprehensive analysis of EGFR-mutant abundance and its effect on efficacy of EGFR TKIs in advanced NSCLC with EGFR mutations. Journal of Thoracic Oncology. 2017;**12**(9):1388-1397

[85] Tan DSW, Chong FT, Leong HS, Toh SY, Lau DP, Kwang XL, et al. Long noncoding RNA EGFR-AS1 mediates epidermal growth factor receptor addiction and modulates treatment response in squamous cell carcinoma. Nature Medicine. 2017;**23**(10):1167-1175

[86] Venturutti L, Cordo Russo RI, Rivas MA, Mercogliano MF, Izzo F, Oakley RH, et al. MiR-16 mediates trastuzumab and lapatinib response in ErbB-2-positive breast and gastric cancer via its novel targets CCNJ and FUBP1. Oncogene. 2016;**35**(48):6189-6202

[87] Zhou CX, Wang CL, Yu AL, Wang QY, Zhan MN, Tang J, et al. MiR-630 suppresses breast cancer progression by targeting metadherin. Oncotarget. 2016;7(2):1288-1299

[88] Chen WX, Zhang ZG, Ding ZY, Liang HF, Song J, Tan XL, et al. MicroRNA-630 suppresses tumor metastasis through the TGF-β-miR-630-Slug signaling pathway and correlates inversely with poor prognosis in hepatocellular carcinoma. Oncotarget. 2016;7(16):22674-22686

[89] Zhao JJ, Chen PJ, Duan RQ, Li KJ, Wang YZ, Li Y. miR-630 functions as a tumor oncogene in renal cell carcinoma. Archives of Medical Science. 2016;**12**(3):473-478

Chapter 5

Cancer Management by Tyrosine Kinase Inhibitors: Efficacy, Limitation, and Future Strategies

Venice Wing Tung Ho, Hor Yue Tan, Ning Wang and Yibin Feng

Abstract

Tyrosine kinase inhibitors are taking up an increasingly significant role in treating cancers. There are different types of TKIs currently used in clinical settings. However, TKI-associated limitations such as resistance and adverse effects are frequently reported. In this chapter, we would comprehensively review the clinical efficacy of current TKIs using the currently available clinical trial data. Significant limitations of TKIs on cancer treatment will be further summarized and discussed. The strategies on overcoming the limitations of TKIs to maximize their clinical effectiveness and efficiency, such as complementary use of Chinese medicine or development of novel TKIs, will be proposed. In conclusion, an overall picture of the clinical use and limitation of the current TKIs will be drawn and the prospective development in overcoming the limitations will be discussed. Evaluation of clinical efficacy of TKIs, evaluation of limitations of TKIs, strategies in overcoming the limitations of TKIs, and conclusion (including prospective development of TKIs) are discussed below.

Keywords: tyrosine kinase inhibitors, targeted therapy, cancer management, clinical efficacy, limitations, future strategies

1. Introduction

The development of tyrosine kinase inhibitors (TKIs) is revolutionary in treating cancers, as they act much more specifically toward malignant cells when compared to conventional cytotoxic chemotherapy [1]. In the past two decades, a plenty of novel compounds under this category have been discovered and are taking up an increasingly significant role in cancer treatment, especially for metastatic carcinomas. Many are proven with great efficacy. They showed significantly better results in progress-free survival rate with fewer side effects [1]. Looking back at the short but eventful history of this drug class, this book chapter intends to do an evaluation on clinical efficacy and effectiveness of TKIs, basing on the currently available clinical trial data. Significant limitations of TKIs on cancer treatment will be further summarized and discussed. Finally, strategies in overcoming the limitations will be proposed. With an overall picture of clinical use and limitations of current TKIs, prospective developmental directions will then be discussed.

IntechOpen

Tyrosine kinases are a subclass of protein kinases, which are enzymes that catalyze the transfer of gamma phosphate group from a nucleoside triphosphate donor (e.g., ATP) to targeted proteins, hence resulting in a conformational change of the protein, which alters its function [2]. Tyrosine kinases are frequently involved in the cellular response to various growth factors, cytokines, and hormones (e.g., EGF, PDGF, VEGF, ABL, and JAK) [3, 4]. These molecules are, in many cases, responsible for the various mechanisms of tumor growth such as cell growth, cell proliferation, stromal growth, angiogenesis, and tissue invasion [4, 5]. In neoplasms, there are often gene mutations resulting in activation of the above pathways [6, 7]. It could be an excessive expression of growth factors/hormones, an excessive expression of their receptors (i.e., increased sensitivity to receptor tyrosine kinases), or intrinsic activation of tyrosine kinases receptors, etc. [7]. Thus, by inhibiting them, we may be able to control or even regress tumor growth.

Tyrosine kinases inhibitors (TKIs) inhibit these growth factor signaling pathways by various mechanisms. They compete with ATP, substrate or for sites for dimerization, and could also act allosterically [8]. By targeting these mutated pathways, TKIs are able to act specifically to cells with malignant changes and disrupt their malignant growth without causing much disturbance to other physiological functioning.

Imatinib was the first tyrosine kinase inhibitor developed, and also the first to be approved by the U.S. Food and Drug administration (FDA) in May 2001. It was approved initially for the use on patients with chronic myeloid leukemia. Shortly after, other tyrosine kinase inhibitors are discovered. There are currently at least 26 FDA-approved tyrosine kinase inhibitors [9] and more going down the pipeline. TKIs were initially only used as second-/third-line therapies, but nowadays, it is increasingly used as primary therapy, especially in selected patients with known mutations.

Tyrosine kinase inhibitors can be classified according to their acting target [10]. Major target classes include BCR-ABLTKIs (e.g., imatinib, dasatinib, and nilotinib), EGFR TKIs (e.g., gefitinib and erlotinib), and VEGFR TKIs (e.g., sunitinib and sorafenib) [10]. Another way to classify them would however be according to their generations. There are up to three, and even four, generations of TKIs. They differ not only by the period they are discovered, but also by their working mechanisms. The first-generation TKIs (e.g., imatinib and gefitinib) are reversible/competitive inhibitors (mostly ATP-competitive inhibitors) and are mostly single-targeted, whereas the second-generation TKIs (e.g., afatinib and dasatinib) and other newer generations of TKIs (e.g., osimertinib) are mostly irreversible/covalent binding and multitargeted [11]. Comparison of approaches used in first and newer generations will be made in later sections.

When compared to traditional chemotherapy and radiation therapy, which simply targets fast-growing cells, TKIs, along with many other targeted drugs, have a much higher specificity toward tumor cells. Thus, they provide a broader therapeutic window with less general toxicity. They are taking up a large role in treating cancers by showing significant improvements in progression-free survival rate and tolerability in patients.

2. Evaluation of clinical efficacy/effectiveness of TKIs

Numerous studies have been conducted to evaluate the clinical efficacy and effectiveness of TKIs. Different TKIs are found to have different clinical performances on different cancers. Most of them showed significant efficacy, especially in improving progression-free survival (PFS), when used as first-line or non–first-line therapies. Therefore, a lot of studies are trying to expand the use of these TKIs to other cancers, yet results are not always promising. However, overall survival was not improved in many cases. A lot of the studies discovered a high percentage of users progressing to drug resistance eventually. In the following, the clinical efficacy and effectiveness of a number of TKIs will be discussed individually. And in the end of this section, a brief comparison is drawn.

2.1 Clinical efficacy/effectiveness of first-generation TKIs

2.1.1 Imatinib (BCR-ABL TKIs)

Imatinib is an orally administered small molecule tyrosine kinase inhibitor, which inhibits tyrosine kinases, specifically BCR-ABL, c-KIT, and PDGFRA [12]. Its marketing name is Gleevec (USA) or Glivec (Europe/Australia), also referred to as CGP57148B or STI571 in some literature [13]. It was invented in 1990s and first approved by FDA in 2001. It has been a huge success and was a revolutionary discovery in combating cancer. Up till today, Imatinib is well known for its efficacy with CML and GIST, and other tumors. A summary on its clinical efficacies will be provided as follows:

2.1.1.1 Chronic myeloid leukemia (CML)

Imatinib is first developed against chronic myeloid leukemia (CML). CML is characterized by the presence of a Philadelphia chromosome [14], which is a product of reciprocal translocation between chromosome 9 and 22. BCL-ABL tyrosine kinase is overexpressed in these CML patients and is a driving force for leukemogenesis [15]. By inhibiting the BCL-ABL tyrosine kinase, Imatinib is found to be able to control the disease effectively. Imatinib has proven significant clinical efficacy and effectiveness, both as a single agent or in combination therapy in chronic phase as well as accelerated phase/blast crisis in CML.

Imatinib, as a single agent, outperformed combined chemotherapy and interferon therapy with major cytogenic response induced in 87.1% (vs. 34.7%) at 18 months [16]. Imatinib also showed significant superiority, when combined with chemotherapy, against the combination of interferon therapy and chemotherapy. In a well-known International Randomized Study (IRIS) on 1106 newly diagnosed CML patients, complete hematological response was induced in 95.3% patients and complete cytogenic response in 73.8% patients [17]. The patients have an overall low risk of progressing to accelerated phase/blast crisis, and overall survival rate at 8 years remained as high as 85% [18] exceeding the reported survival rates in all previous CML therapies. Other studies trying to combine imatinib with other therapies, including chemotherapy and IFN, showed that MCR/CCR did tend to occur earlier, for example, rate of MCR at 3 months was 70% compared to 60% when combining imatinib with cytarabine. Yet the gap seemed to close after 12 months, with 84 and 83%, respectively. Combinations have however also resulted in more severe side effects, and are thus in general not preferred [19]. Other studies echo their results and have shown that imatinib in combination with chemotherapy does not display superiority against imatinib as a monotherapy in CML-chronic phase, but instead yielded more toxicity [20, 21].

Imatinib is proved effective in accelerated phase/blast crisis as well [19, 22]. However, there are also studies reporting that its effects are only transient, and can only produce palliative function to those patients at this stage [23]. Acquired resistance developed in a large portion of the cases treated with imatinib. Acquired resistance was defined as a progression of disease or loss of response with a 5- to 10-fold increase in BCL-ABL transcripts. These patients are subsequently treated with higher dosage of imatinib, or a second-generation BCR-ABL TKI. Yet, allogenic hematopoietic cell transplantation remains the ultimate solution.

Response rate of imatinib in unselected CML patients is high only due to the high occurrence (91%) of the presence of Philadelphia chromosome [24, 25]. Its clinical efficacy in Philadelphia chromosome negative patients is however very low.

2.1.1.2 Gastrointestinal stromal tumors (GIST)

Gastrointestinal stromal tumor is the most common neoplasm of the mesenchymal cells of the digestive system and is thought to arise from the interstitial cells of Cajal [26]. C-KIT and PDGFRA tyrosine kinase mutations are present in a vast majority (85%) of these tumors [27–29]. Imatinib is able to inhibit the mutant C-KIT and PDGFRA tyrosine kinases. Imatinib has high efficacy against GIST in patients with these two mutations, both as an adjuvant therapy after surgery in non-metastatic GISTs, and as a palliative treatment for advanced non-resectable GISTs. For primary resectable GISTs, recurrence rate after surgery is extremely high. Studies have found that adjuvant therapy of imatinib can prolong relapse free survival (RFS), especially in those patients with great risks of relapse [30, 31]. Absolute relapse rate was 19 vs. 47% in imatinib treated patients and non-treated patients, respectively [30, 32]. Other studies have shown that imatinib displays similar promising results in GISTs in advanced stages as well. Approximately 80% of GIST patients with advanced disease receive some benefit from imatinib therapy [33], with median overall survival of 57 months, compared to 18 in chemotherapy. Yet, a significant proportion eventually became resistant with a median time to progression of 2 years [33]. Primary resistance was found in around 12% of the patients [34]. It was also found that, higher dosage of Imatinib showed no superiority over lower dosage [35, 36]. In GIST patients, side effects arose in 99% of the case [37]. The most common adverse events were diarrhea (29% of patients), nausea (27%), eyelid edema (23%), peripheral edema (22%), muscle cramps (15%), and fatigue (13%) [38]. Luckily, most patients found the side effects tolerable [37].

2.1.1.3 Others

Imatinib was also approved by the FDA and has now become the first-line treatment for patients with Philadelphia chromosome positive acute lymphoblastic leukemia (Ph + ALL), which accounts for approximately 30% of all ALL cases [39]. Patients treated with imatinib early are found to have higher overall survival, event-free survival, and relapse-free survival [40]. Studies have also justified the efficacy of imatinib in dermatofibrosarcoma protuberans [41, 42], chronic eosinophilic leukemia [43], systemic mastocytosis [44, 45], aggressive fibromatosis [46], malignant melanoma [47], AIDS-related Kaposi's sarcoma [48], chordoma [49, 50], recurrent epithelial ovarian cancer [51], and anaplastic thyroid cancer [52]. The use of imatinib in these cancers is not yet approved, but lots of clinical trials have already been conducted and their use in the future is expected.

2.1.1.4 Tolerability of side effects

Clinical trials have shown that the side effects of imatinib are generally well-tolerated by the patients. Common side effects include edema, rash, nausea, diarrhea, muscle cramps, and more severely, myelosuppression [53]. Luckily, most side effects were mild to moderate, and in more than 95% of the patients, side effects could be managed with standard concomitant treatments [38].

2.1.2 Gefitinib and erlotinib (EGFR TKIs)

Gefitinib (Iressa, ZD1839) and erlotinib (Tarceva, OSI774) are the two first-generation EGFR-TKIs and are used mostly against non-small cell lung cancer (NSCLC), which accounts for 85% of all lung cancers [54]. As competitive antagonists of the ATP-binding site of EGFR, gefitinib and erlotinib were approved by the FDA in May 2003 and November 2004, respectively. As many cancers involve the hyperactivity of EGFRs, numerous studies have been conducted on drug repurposing of these two TKIs.

2.1.2.1 Non-small cell lung cancer

Gefitinib and Erlotinib are most established in treating non-small cell lung cancer (NSCLC) and are currently the first-line treatment for EGFR-mutated NSCLC patients [55]. EGFR mutations are commonly found in NSCLC patients, particularly in Asian populations, female gender, and nonsmokers [56, 57]. EGFR mutations are associated with the activation of antiapoptotic pathways as well as proliferation induction, thus leading to uncontrolled growth of cells. Among all the types of NSCLC, adenocarcinoma takes up the largest proportion, and is also the most commonly associated with EGFR mutations. Gefitinib was initially approved against NSCLC, but was then withdrawn from the market due to various studies showing its lack of benefit in overall survival in unselected patients. However, it was later found that EGFR mutation is a huge positive predicting factor for drug response to gefitinib, and was thus approved again. Gefitinib has well established clinical efficacy against advanced NSCLC when compared to chemotherapy [58, 59]. Progression-free survival was 10.8 vs. 5.4 months and mean overall survival was 30.5 vs. 23.6 months [59]. Combination of gefitinib with chemotherapy showed no superiority over gefitinib monotherapy [60]. Similarly, Erlotinib showed significant superiority over chemotherapy in EGFR mutation positive advanced NSCLC (PFS 13.1 vs. 4.6 months) [61]. However, its overall survival was reported to be lower than that of chemotherapy (24.68 vs. 26.16 months) [62]. Erlotinib plus chemotherapy is superior to chemotherapy alone with an improved PFS but not OS [63]. A meta-analysis revealed that the efficacy between gefitinib and erlotinib are comparable with erlotinib reported of more adverse drug effects [64].

Clinical effectiveness in unselected NSCLC patients were low as the frequency of EGFR gene mutation is 47.9% in Asians but only 19.2% in Western patients [65]. About only 10–35% of the NSCLC patients have EGFR mutations which are sensitive to the EGFR TKIs [66]. Progression-free survival in rare EGFR mutations was also lower than that of common EGFR mutations, yet the overall survival was similar [67, 68].

2.1.2.2 Other

There are currently some researches conducted on the use of gefitinib and erlotinib on other cancers, yet most are currently not approved yet. Gefitinib is reported to show effect on pancreatic cancer [69] and is approved to treat metastatic pancreatic cancer in combination with chemotherapy in 2005. The effects of gefitinib and erlotinib on other cancers are also being investigated, such as nasopharyngeal cancer [70], gastric cancer [71], esophageal cancer [72], cervical cancer [73], renal cell carcinoma [74], and hepatocellular carcinoma [75]. Yet most studies are still in preclinical stages, and those limited clinical trials were often with disappointing results.

2.1.2.3 Tolerability of side effects

Gefitinib has better tolerability than many cytotoxic drugs [76]. Acne-like rash was reported as the most common side effect, others include nausea, diarrhea, anorexia, stomatitis, dehydration, etc. Side effects were in general well-tolerated and few withdraw from gefitinib due to intolerability [76]. Erlotinib is in general well tolerated as well. Yet it was reported to have more severe side effects than that of gefitinib and was more frequently involved with dosage reduction due to side effect intolerance [77]. Significantly higher rates and severity of skin rash, nausea, vomiting, fatigue, and stomatitis were also reported.

2.1.3 Sunitinib and sorafenib (VEGFR TKIs)

Sunitinib (Sutent, SU11248) and sorafenib (Nexavar) are first-generation VEGFR-TKIs and are well established in the use against renal cell carcinoma (RCC) and hepatocellular carcinoma (HCC), respectively. The VEGF family are frequently overexpressed in various solid tumors and bind to vascular endothelium and induce angiogenesis. Sunitinib and sorafenib are both multitarget ATP-competitive TKIs. Sunitinib inhibits tyrosine kinases such as VEGFR2, PDGFRβ, KIT, RET, CSF1R, and FLT3. Sorafenib inhibits tyrosine kinases including VEGFRs, PDGFRs, B-RAF, MEK, and ERK. They are both FDA approved for RCC, GIST and RCC, HCC, respectively. Their clinical efficacies are discussed below.

2.1.3.1 RCC

VEGF overexpression and high vascularization is a common feature of RCC. Both sunitinib and sorafenib were approved for renal cell carcinoma as first- and second-line therapies. Sunitinib was approved for metastatic RCC (mRCC) in 2006 after a phase III trial showing its superiority over IFN therapy [78]. Sunitinib displayed well clinical efficacy and effectiveness with median OS 26.4 months and PFS 11.0 months, especially in clear cell RCC, compared to OS 21.8 months in IFN therapy [78]. However, study also showed that median PFS and OS are not significantly different in poor-risk group [79]. Finally, a large scaled clinical trials conducted on unselected heterogeneous RCC patients confirmed the effectiveness of sunitinib [80]. Combination of sunitinib with chemotherapy was not explored after phase I trials showing its poor safety profile [81]. Trials combining sunitinib with other therapies have also shown no improved efficacy, yet increased toxicity [82]. On the other hand, Sorafenib was also proven to have high clinical efficacy against mRCC, both as first- and second-line therapy [83]. It was found to prolong PFS when compared to placebo after the failure of immunotherapy [84]. Yet there is no statistically significant difference in OS. Studies comparing efficacy of sunitinib and sorafenib showed no significant difference, with sorafenib slightly superior in elderly patients [85]. Sequence of use of sunitinib and sorafenib also has no significant difference [86].

2.1.3.2 HCC

Preclinical studies have demonstrated that MEK and ERK pathways play a role in hepatocellular carcinoma [87]. VEGF pathway also plays a significant role in angiogenesis in HCC [88]. This provides a window of opportunity of prolonging survival through TKIs targeting these pathways, including sorafenib. For unresectable HCC, especially in cases where potential curative methods or transarterial chemoembolization (TACE) are not available, Sorafenib is highly recommended as it demonstrates high clinical efficacy [89]. Sorafenib was reported with 3 months longer in median overall survival (10.7 vs. 7.9) when compared to placebo [90]. Yet there was no significant difference in the median progression time to symptomatic progression [91]. Sorafenib, when combined with chemotherapy, also showed superiority over chemotherapy alone, with PFS 6.0 vs. 2.7 months and OS 13.7 vs. 6.5 months [92]. Yet it has poor effectiveness in generalized HCC patients and many argue that its efficacy is questionable [93].

2.1.3.3 GIST

Sunitinib is used against GIST as well and has been approved for usage following failure/intolerance of imatinib in 2006 [94]. The median time to progression was 27.3 weeks compared to 6.4 weeks in placebo [95]. There was no overall survival benefit of sunitinib over placebo, but the results were not reliable due to crossing over of placebo patients to sorafenib group. Studies have been conducted to modify the patient selection procedure in attempt to further raise its effectiveness, but are all in vain [96]. On the other hand, sorafenib also showed certain efficacy toward GIST. Yet its efficacy was lower than that of imatinib, and was thus only used as third/fourth line, after failure of initial therapy [97].

2.1.3.4 Differentiated thyroid cancer (DTC)

Sorafenib is also approved for use against advanced thyroid cancer which are resistant to radioactive iodine. Prior to the discovery of sorafenib, there was no effective treatment for this group of patients and overall survival was poor [98]. With sorafenib, a phase III trial showed that their PFS is greatly improved when compared to placebo (10.8 vs. 5.8 months) and thus provides a new treatment option for radioactive iodine resistant advanced DTC patients [99].

2.1.3.5 Tolerability of side effects

Compared to other TKIs, the tolerability of sunitinib is lower. Adverse events of any grade are reported in up to 95% of patients with one-third drug interruption due to intolerability in metastatic RCC [100]. Most common grade 3/4 adverse events include thrombocytopenia (10%), fatigue (9%), and asthenia, neutropenia and hand foot mouth syndrome (each 7%) [80]. It is commonly associated with various side effects including hypertension, hypothyroidism, diarrhea, fatigue, and nausea. Therefore, studies have recommended a special schedule for the administration for this reason, with 2-week drug use followed by a 1-week drug holiday alternatively, which offers a similar efficacy but with higher tolerability [101–103]. Sorafenib has a slightly better safety profile [104]. Safety profile agrees with what is previously reported, with hand–foot skin reaction (58.0%), lipase elevation (57.3%), and diarrhea (42.7%) as the most frequent drug-related adverse events. Neither unknown adverse event nor cumulative toxicity was observed over the long-term use of sorafenib [105]. Yet intolerability remains one of its greatest limitations.

2.2 Clinical efficacy/effectiveness of second-generation TKIs

2.2.1 Dasatinib, nilotinib, bosutinib, and radotinib (BCR-ABL TKIs)

Following the success of Imatinib, many second-generation TKIs targeting BCR-ABL have also been developed. These include dasatinib, nilotinib, bosutinib, and radotinib, and also a few more that will not be included in this discussion, including

ON012380, MK0457, PHA739358, etc. They are much more potent than imatinib and showed promising efficacy in treating patients who have failed imatinib treatment [106].

Dasatinib (Sprycel, DB01254) was the first FDA approved among them and is a dual Src and ABL kinase inhibitor. Besides binding to these two kinases, it also has inhibitory effect on PDGFRβ, c-KIT, and EPHA2 [107]. By targeting more kinases than those of imatinib, dasatinib is able to tackle multiple types of resistant mechanisms against imatinib, including secondary BCR-ABL mutation, alternative Src signaling pathway activation, and multidrug resistance gene overexpression. Study showed durable results of treatment with dasatinib following imatinib. Imatinib resistant/intolerant patients showed early (3–6 months) complete cytogenic response and major molecular response, and were associated with better PFS and OS rates [108, 109]. When compared to imatinib as first-line treatment to newly diagnosed CML, dasatinib showed even better response. It was able to achieve higher percentage of complete cytogenic response and major molecular response with a higher rate [110].

Nilotinib (Tasigna, AMN107), on the other hand, is more structurally similar to imatinib, but is 20–50 folds more potent. Nilotinib was another huge success. It was able to induce complete hematological response in 92% of the patients who were resistant/intolerant to imatinib [111]. Similarly, it was also found to be superior as first-line treatment than imatinib for newly diagnosed Ph + CML [112]. Both Dasatinib and Nilotinib are found to give similar results in large community settings as well. When compared to first-generation TKI imatinib, dasatinib and nilotinib performed significantly better as first-line treatment to newly diagnosed CML patients. They achieve higher Complete Cytogenic Response (CCyR) or Major Molecular Response (MMR) at 6, 12, and 18 months, respectively. By 12 months, 61% patients achieved CCyR or MMR compared to only 38% treated with imatinib. Time to MMR is also significantly higher in dasatinib and nilotinib than imatinib [113].

Bosutinib (Bosulif, SKI606) was initially approved in CML-AP/BC, and is later expanded to CML-CP. Trials prove improved rates of MMR at 12 months when compared to imatinib (47.2 vs. 36.9%) [114]. Soon it was also used as first-line therapy against CML.

Radotinib (Supect, IY5511) also showed significant superiority over imatinib. With minimum 12 months follow-up, radotinib demonstrated significantly higher and faster rates of CCyR and MMR than imatinib in patients with newly diagnosed CML-CP [115].

2.2.1.1 *Tolerability of side effects*

The second-generation BCR-ABL TKIs seem to have significantly higher efficacy than imatinib. Yet, their side effects are also more severe than that of imatinib. This is likely due to the increased potency as well as multi-targeting of the drugs. For example, when comparing bosutinib to imatinib, patients taking bosutinib have higher rates of increased liver enzyme values (24 vs. 4%), thrombocytopenia (13.8 vs. 5.7%), neutropenia (6.7 vs. 12.1%), and diarrhea (7.8 vs. <1%). 77.9% patients experienced severe Grade 3/4 adverse events and 24% patients had to discontinue bosutinib therapy due to emergence of adverse events in a study [116]. Radotinib's side effects are also more severe than that of imatinib. Grade 3/4 ALT/AST elevations caused 68% dosage reduction/interruption in radotinib patients, but only 19% in imatinib patients.

2.2.2 *Afatinib and dacomitinib (EGFR TKIs)*

Second-generation EGFR TKIs are irreversible inhibitors and are designed to target other ErbB family members, including HER2, to have more potent inhibition.

They target not only the T790M mutation of EGFR, but also other EGFR-activating mutations as well as wild-type EGFR [117].

Afatinib (Gilotrif, BIBW2992) is an irreversible inhibitor for the ERBB family, including HER1(EGFR), HER2, and HER4. Studies have proven that afatinib was effective in prolonging PFS when compared to chemotherapy (median PFS 11.1 vs. 6.9 months) [118]. When compared to erlotinib, afatinib can also significantly increase PFS by 18%, improve OS by 19% and improve disease control rate (51 vs. 40%) in NSCLC patients after failure of chemotherapy. It was eventually approved by FDA as another first-line therapy for NSCLC.

Dacomitinib (PF299804) is also an irreversible inhibitor of the ERBB family, including HER1(EGFR), HER2 and 4. It is currently still in the preregistration stage and is not approved yet in any country. Findings have shown superiority over gefitinib: PFS 14.7 months with dacomitinib vs. 9.2 months with gefitinib as first-line therapy [119, 120].

Second-generation EGFR-TKIs exhibit many dose-limiting toxicities, mainly skin and GI toxicities, as they inhibit WT-EGFRs as well [117].

2.2.3 Pazopanib, tivozanib, axitinib, and regorafenib (VEGFR TKIs)

Pazopanib (Votrient, GW786034B) was compared to sunitinib and showed superiority. It was shown to significantly improve PFS when compared to placebo in both treatment naïve and cytokine-pretreated patients of RCC [121]. Similar to the first-generation VEGFR-TKIs, Pazopanib inhibits a large number of pathways, including VEGFR, c-KIT, FGFR, PDGFRβ. The lack of specificity accounts for its multiple side effects. Yet, its tolerability is higher than that of sorafenib and sunitinib [122, 123].

Tivozanib and axitinib on the contrary, are well-known for their higher selectivity. Tivozanib (Fotivda, AV-951) is highly selective for VEGFR. In a study conducted on metastatic RCC, Tivozanib outperformed sorafenib as first-line treatment in prolonging PFS [124]. The study revealed that Tivozanib improved PFS in RCC by 3 months (30%) when compared to sorafenib, yet has an inferior overall survival [124, 125]. For this reason, it is unable to obtain approval from FDA. It was however approved by the European Medicines Agency (EMA). Axitinib (Inlyta, AG13736) is also highly selective for VEGFR. Axitinib was proved to be better than sorafenib in treating RCCs by giving longer PFS (6.8 vs. 4.7 months) in pretreated patients and are thus approved as second-line use.

Regorafenib (STIVARGA) is approved by the FDA in 2012 for its use in metastatic colorectal cancer (mCRC) and GIST. Regorafenib monotherapy was found to significantly improve OS (6.4 vs. 5.0 months) in mCRC when compared to placebo following failure of standard therapy [126]. Soon after, its efficacy in GIST was also found. A clinical trial compared patients treated with regorafenib monotherapy vs. placebo after acquiring resistance against imatinib and sunitinib [127]. PFS was way higher in regorafenib group (4.8 vs. 0.9 months) and is thus approved by the FDA. OS was however not determined as the patients in the placebo group were crossed over to the regorafenib group after disease progression.

2.2.3.1 Tolerability of side effects

Their tolerability is significantly better than sorafenib, especially with tivozanib. Drug dosage reduction due to intolerance was 11.6% in tivozanib, but 42.8% in sorafenib [125].

2.3 Clinical efficacy/effectiveness of third-generation TKIs

2.3.1 Ponatinib (BCR-ABL TKIs)

Ponatinib (Iclusig, IY5511) is a multitargeted TKI including BCR-ABL. It was specifically designed for T315I mutation-caused imatinib resistance. Studies have proven its high clinical efficacy of inducing cytogenic response in 66% CML-CP patients, which include all of the T315I mutation positive patients. Yet, in generalized CML-CP patients, ponatinib did not show significantly superior efficacy than the previous second- and first-generation TKIs [128]. Thus, it is suggested for first-line use only in the setting of detected T315I mutation, otherwise, merely as a second-line treatment following first- and second-generation TKIs.

2.3.1.1 Tolerability of side effects

Treatment-related side effects are moderately significant with ponatinib. Common adverse events include rash (47%), abdominal pain (46%), thrombocytopenia (46%), headache (43%), dry skin (42%), and constipation (41%). It is however associated with a severe adverse event, which is arterial occlusive events (AOE), which occurred in a cumulative of 31% patients.

2.3.2 Osimertinib (EGFR)

Due to the limited efficacy in tackling T790M resistance of EGFR of the second-generation TKIs, the third generation of EGFR-TKIs has been discovered. Third generation works significantly better against the T790M-mutated EGFR while sparing the wild-type EGFRs, making them very mutant selective. Various third-generation EGFR-TKIs are currently under clinical trials, including osimertinib, PF06747775, YH5448, avitinib, rociletinib, etc. Of them all, osimertinib is the only currently approved drug.

Osimertinib (Tagrisso, AZD9291) is a very promising third-generation EGFR-TKI. It is able to tackle gefitinib/erlotinib acquired resistance through T790M, exon 19 and 21, which accounts for a large portion of acquired resistant cases. In a FLAURA study, Osimertinib was compared to first-line EGFR-TKIs (erlotinib and gefitinib) as first line therapy [129]. It showed significantly higher efficacy against EGFR-mutated patients, with PFS 18.9 vs. 10.2 months. An extra feature of osimertinib is its ability to penetrate the blood-brain barrier and tackle patients with brain metastasis as well. CNS progression was lower in patients treated with osimertinib (6 vs. 15%). There is not yet data available on comparing overall survival between the two, yet osimertinib showed a trend of superiority. At 18 months of the FLAURA study, 83% of the patients in the osimertinib group were still alive vs. 71% in the first-generation EGFR-TKI group. Most third-generation EGFR-TKIs combat the T790M EGFR resistance mechanism selectively. Yet, the other 50% resistant mechanisms remain a challenge.

2.3.2.1 Tolerability of side effects

Side effects of third-generation EGFR-TKIs are rather mild and tolerable. Side effects of Osimertinib commonly include rash, nausea, and diarrhea. Grade 3 or 4 adverse events occurred in 24% of the patients, but only 2% of the patients required a dosage reduction, and only 4% discontinuation. However, there are also studies which disagree. In the FLAURA study, rate of permanent discontinuation due to adverse events of osimertinib was 13%. Yet it is still lower than that of those receiving first-generation EGFR-TKIs, which was 18% [129].

2.4 Comparison

2.4.1 Newer generations perform better than first generation

Viewed as a whole, TKIs of the later generations tend to outperform the first generation in terms of efficacy. This is mainly because the newer generations tend to target multiple pathways and also provide a more potent irreversible inhibition. This allows them to be effective in both first-line setting, as well as combatting heterogeneous resistant mechanisms arisen. Yet, their downside is the occurrence of more severe side effects. The third-generation TKIs thus aim at targeting multiple pathways while sparing physiological functions, e.g., third-generation EGFR-TKIs. VEGFR-TKIs are the exceptions. Their first-generation TKIs are multitargeted, and their newer generation TKIs are more specific, and thus offer a higher tolerability. Studies on newer generations of TKIs delineate promising results on both their efficacy as a potential first-line treatment and as a second-line treatment after acquired resistance of the initial therapy.

2.4.1.1 High efficacy but low effectiveness

Many TKIs seem to show merely improvement in progression-free survival, but not in overall survival rate. These include gefitinib in NSCLC [130], sunitinib, nilotinib and regorafenib in GIST [131], lenvatinib in differentiated thyroid cancer [132], and many other TKIs, regardless of whether they are of newer generations or not. Erlotinib even showed poorer overall survival rate than chemotherapy (24.68 vs. 26.16 months), despite a significantly higher progression-free survival [62]. The potential reasons shall be further discussed.

Response rate of TKIs are low in unselected patients. Various studies have shown that, in the absence of targeted mutation, targeted therapy performed worse than traditional chemotherapy. Presence of targeted mutation is a huge positive predicting factor for good tumor response [133, 134]. Response rate in unselected population is however high in a few cases, for example, in unselected CML patients. This is likely because the vast majority of them carry the same single mutation of BCR-ABL. It is also high in RCC for first-generation TKIs, since the first-generation VEGFR-TKIs are relatively nonspecific, and are able to target multiple mutation mechanisms.

3. Evaluation of limitations of TKIs

3.1 Development of resistance

The development of resistance has always been and will probably always be the greatest problem limiting the use of TKIs. The rate of developing acquired resistance (AR) is extremely high, and appears even to be inevitable in certain diseases. In EGFR-TKI therapy, a study showed the median time for patients developing AR is 8–10 months, and all responding patients developed AR eventually, with the inevitable consequence of disease progression [135, 136]. The case with imatinib is slightly better; around 7–15% is found to have secondary resistance, i.e., disease progression following initial achievement of cytogenic response [137, 138]. And this is the reason why the PFS, despite longer than chemotherapy, is still not very long, with most ranging from a few months to at most a few years, despite their high disease response rate and promptness in controlling the disease. Acquiring resistance and disease progression seem almost inevitable in many cancer lines using TKIs. This phenomenon occurs indiscriminately in all generations of TKIs and is a huge challenge.

The development of resistance comes in many ways, and many researches have been dedicated to finding out the mechanisms of resistance to TKIs. Studies have shown that cancer cells adapt to chronic therapy by through common mechanisms found include secondary mutations of target, activation of alternative signaling pathway, evading immune system and adaptive or cell fate changes, etc. Point mutation at site coding for TK resulting in decreased affinity for the TKI remains the most prevalent mechanism of acquired resistance [139]. Point mutations (esp. T315I mutation) in CML patients are a major cause in AR toward imatinib. Occurrence of these mutations reduces the life expectancy of chronic phase CML patients from 10 years to just 22 months [140]. Exon 20-T790M mutation is found in approximately half of the patients with progressed disease following initial EGFR-TKI use [141]. Any of the ways allow the tumor cells to regain its ability to grow and divide. The heterogeneity of resistance mechanisms poses huge difficulty for a single TKI to produce high response rate following AR to the initial TKI.

Newer generations of TKIs aimed at resolving acquired resistance toward the older generation TKIs. Yet, there are too many different types of resistance mechanisms that could arise between different patients, as discussed. Taking NSCLC AR to erlotinib and gefitinib as an example, AR mechanism could be T790M missense mutation, other secondary mutations of EGFR, MET amplification, HER2 amplification, small cell histological transformation, etc. And up to 30% of the NSCLC patients with AR to first gen TKIs have unknown resistance mechanism [135]. Its heterogeneity makes the development of new generation TKIs, especially one with high tumor response, very hard.

The management of post-TKI disease progression is a new therapeutic challenge. The ways to overcome include using multitargeted approach, in which the TKI is effective against a broad spectrum of resistance mechanisms, or perform genetic tests and learning the specific resistance mechanism of the individual patient and selecting the next TKI. Details are discussed in the next session.

3.2 Complexity and redundancy in tumor pathways and between tumor subclones

Multiple regulatory factors and multiple signaling pathways exist within a tumor, and they each share a role in supporting tumor growth [142]. Many elements of these pathways are redundant, and contribute toward the same function. With all these redundancy, inhibiting one factor or one pathway will often not be sufficient in inhibiting tumor growth [143]. This is part of the reason for the robustness of cancer cells, allowing them to survive through a diversity of treatments. Take angiogenesis as an example. Although VEGF is the most potent stimulatory regulator of angiogenesis, and human cancers often have an overexpression of VEGF, there are also many other stimulatory and inhibitory factors involved, which some are produced by tumor cells and some by the host cells. Therefore, simply administrating a single-target VEGFR-TKIs may not result in significant antiangiogenic effect. Besides, some of the factors, including VEGF, can exist in multiple isoforms, making it even harder to inhibit the angiogenic process [1, 144]. Moreover, many tumors have more than one mutated pathways, for instance, both VEGFR and PDGFR mutation [145]. It is only through multitargeting and combination therapy, or targeting more upstream pathways, could a more significant response be brought about [143]. Simply inhibiting one target is in many cases not effective enough to hinder cell growth.

With technology of next-generation sequencing of patient biopsies, it has been revealed that tumors contain vastly heterogeneous genetic alterations in multiple subclones. This is also called intratumor heterogeneity. This also includes geographical heterogeneity, in which the genetic makeup of metastatic tumors differs from each other as well. As the neoplastic cells divide and undergo DNA replication, the clones are highly prone to genetic mutations, and the mutated cells continue to grow and give rise to their colony of cells. Thus within the same tumor, there could be multiple subclones each with their own variant of DNA makeup. This plays a huge role in the development of resistance toward TKIs. Heterogenic tumor subclones may exhibit different sensitivity toward the TKIs. Some tumors may have primary resistance, and with the TKI acting as the selecting pressure, the resistant subclones are selected and are able to continue growing. This accounts for the high rate of resistance toward TKIs. And research has also proven that high intratumoral heterogeneity predicts poorer prognosis and poorer response to treatment [146].

3.3 Poor patient selection

Low effectiveness of TKIs in studies may be due to poor patient selection. By knowing the mechanism of action of the TKIs, we know well that they could only work in a selected population of tumor cells, which contains the pharmacological target. They do not always work well in unselected populations. There are a certain portion of cancer cell lines which are innately resistant to the TKI therapy administered. In unselected NSCLC patients, only 15 in 58 in Japan and 1 in 61 in USA responded to the gefitinib treatment [147]. This is due to the heterogeneity of mutations of the same cancer in different individuals. This occurs not only with initial therapy option, but also newer generations of TKIs as well as non–first-line TKIs. Response rates of many newly developed EGFR-TKIs, targeting at patients with AR to first-line TKIs, were lower than 10%. These include neratinib, whose response rate is 3% [148] and IPI-504, whose response rate is 4% [148]. Therefore, poor patient selection will greatly limit the effectiveness of TKIs. Mechanisms for patient selection must be developed in order to increase TKI effectiveness in community settings.

3.4 Antagonistic drug interaction

Many studies found that combining TKI with traditional chemotherapy showed no significant benefit, but rather an additive effect of toxicity, resulting in disappointment. Concurrent administration may not be effective due to TKI induced G1 phase cell cycle arrest [149]. Although combination approach is believed to provide better outcome in many cases, practitioners must pay attention to antagonistic drug interactions in order to prevent this from limiting the effectiveness of TKI. Alternating administration schedule is proposed for many combination therapies in order to avoid this problem.

3.5 Side effects

Although TKIs are deemed to be relatively well tolerated, especially when compared to systemic cytotoxic chemotherapy, there are still many cases of side effects limiting the use of this drug. With variations from drug to drug, up to 50% report cases of skin toxicity and folliculitis with TKI use. EGFR TKIs display a broad spectrum of skin and hair adverse effects, including folliculitis, facial hair growth, facial erythema, paronychia, and varying forms of frontal alopecia, whereas VEGFR TKIs are more commonly associated with subungual splinter hemorrhages. Imatinib frequently causes periorbital edema. TKIs produce various hematological side effects (anemia, thrombocytopenia, neutropenia) and extra-hematological side effects, most commonly being edema, nausea, hypothyroidism, vomiting, and diarrhea. Regarding long-term effects, cardiac toxicity with congestive heart failure is discussed in patients receiving imatinib and sunitinib [150]. Adverse events have been reported in the use of sorafenib against HCC, including Hand Foot Skin Reactions (HFSR), hyperbilirubinemia associated with heightened ALT. Adverse effects occurred in up to 40% of differentiated thyroid cancer patients, which are mainly hypertension, diarrhea, asthenia, or fatigue, nausea, decreased weight and appetite. This had resulted in dosage reduction despite good tumor response [151]. About 14% of the patients had to discontinue therapy due to intolerance of adverse events. Severity of side effects was found correlated with specificity of the TKIs. The newer generations are usually multitargeted, and thus yield more severe side effects. Luckily, third generations are more mutant selective, and thus showed improvement in this aspect.

3.6 Lack of follow-up and nonadherence

As TKI is a drug class that has to be administrated over a long period of time, the lack of follow-up during the course of treatment is a problem that could limit the effectiveness. In a study reporting effectiveness of TKIs in CML patients in a community setting, it is found that cytogenetic and molecular response monitoring assessments were conducted less frequently than recommended [113]. Poor monitoring may result in delay in adjustments in treatment plan. On the other hand, TKIs are mostly administrated orally, which may pose a challenge in patient adherence. Poor patient compliance plays a role in increasing rates of acquired resistance to TKIs. It is found that, as the treatment progresses, those with higher adherence did achieve better results in achieving CCyR and MMR [113]. While adherence to TKIs is critical in achieving durable responses, it is surprising that merely 56% patients in a study of 229 CML patients adhere to their dosage (which is defined as ^{3}90% adherence) [113].

3.7 Financial burden on patients

There have been numerous studies conducted on cost-effectiveness of TKIs. But most work on merely the comparison between different TKIs or compare TKIs with other treatment. As TKIs are in many occasions not covered by the public health system, they are usually self-funded, unless the patient is covered by insurance, has successfully applied for external funding or is enrolled in a clinical trial. The average per person total cost of treatment with branded imatinib is (79,000 USD/year) and even higher for dasatinib and nilotinib (87,000–92,000 USD/year) [152]. The humongous financial burden complicates the patients' decision in drug choice. It may also affect their choice of continuation of treatment. Studies have shown that high costs of TKIs even lead to a delay in treatment for many patients with leukemia [153]. Some patients may resort to generic TKIs, which quality may not be always consistently good. For example, a study showed that generic Imatinib show suboptimal efficacy when compared to branded imatinib as first-line therapy in CML [154].

4. Strategies in overcoming the limitations of TKIs

Plenty studies have been coming up with all sorts of strategies in overcoming the limitations of TKIs. The big direction is to develop new inhibitors, use a combination approach, and improve patient selection.

4.1 Development of new inhibitors: specific approach and multitargeted approach

Following post-TKI disease progression, continuing the use of the initial TKI therapy does not improve PFS [155]. There is thus a desperate need for new treatment options, or new TKIs. Various studies are working on drugs available for use after acquired resistance. A large number of new TKIs are working their way down the pipeline, in preclinical studies and clinical studies, a lot of which are very promising. The new inhibitors are either very specific toward a certain type of acquired mutation, or multitargeted to inhibit a broader spectrum of pathways, in order to overcome resistance.

With next-generation sequencing, we are able to identify the specific mutations and design molecules that specifically target them. The mutation mechanisms are however vast in diversity. Taking acquired resistance to imatinib in GIST as an example, in a study, among the 15 patients who acquired resistance to imatinib, 7 were found with secondary mutation at the KIT target, 6 of which occurred at the exon 17 (three were N822K, two were D820Y and one was Y823D) [156]. Luckily we were also able to identify some more common ones, e.g., T790M mutation in EGFR-TKI AR. One of the strategies is thus to develop drugs that target these mutations specifically. To facilitate this, however, there should be more research on mechanisms of acquired resistance against TKIs in different cancers. However, this would also be a very costly method.

Another approach of new inhibitors, also a more practical approach, would be the multi-targeted approach, as well as the inhibiting of upstream pathways. As stated previously, the vast heterogeneity within tumor subclones and the redundancy of cancer cell signaling pathways poses a huge challenge for targeted therapies. One of the strategies regarding is to have multiple targets. Network model suggests that partial inhibition of multiple targets may exhibit better effect than complete inhibition of a single target [157]. This has been the trend in many newly developed drugs. Many studies agree that multi-targeted TKIs should perform better than single-targeted ones in terms of efficacy and tumor response rate [145, 158–160]. When targeting a single molecule, the cancer cells can easily adapt and bend around the hindered pathway by activation of alternative pathways. By interacting with multiple targets simultaneously, it leaves less chance for cancer cells to do so [159, 161]. Multitargeted approach also eliminates the malignant cells faster as they inhibit multiple pathways, inhibiting the cancer cells at multiple levels.

Identifying convergent resistance mechanisms or targeting upstream pathways enables us to achieve something similar. Despite the large number of resistance mechanisms, a lot of them converge on reactivation of the driving pathway. For example, in BRAF-mutant melanomas, 89% of resistance mechanisms lie within the MAPK pathway [162]. Identifying these convergent resistance mechanisms could allow us to combat acquired resistance more effortlessly.

However, the multi-targeted approach is also with more severe adverse effects than the single-targeted [158]. It is thus important to be able to identify the suitable set of targets, which allows us to be specific enough to act selectively at the tumor cells only, not the normal body cells, yet not specific enough to prevent cancer cells from acquiring resistance too easily. Luckily, we are equipped with newer tools, including the network pharmacology approach, to aid us in the design of these new drugs [157].

4.2 Combination therapy

Combination approach with a similar mindset when that of developing multitargeted TKIs, it is believed that a combination of therapies would leave less chance for selection of resistant subclones, which allows the tumor to acquire resistance.

TKIs treatment could potentially combine with many different treatments. Many studies have already been conducted on the combination of TKIs with conventional therapies, including chemotherapy, radiation therapy, interferon therapy, etc. A study showed that combination of standard-dose imatinib and IF-therapy yielded better results than standard-dose or high-dose imatinib alone, as well as standard-dose imatinib combined with chemotherapy [21, 163]. Icotinib, an EGFR-TKI is proved to improve radiosensitivity in lung cancer in vitro and in vivo, thus possibly allowing better radiotherapy effects [164]. They are extensively studied and are in many cases already put to clinical practice.

A TKI could also be combined with another TKI. For example, dual EGFR blockade by first and third-generation EGFR TKI combinations [165]. Or dual ALK and EGFR target inhibition in ALK translocated NSCLC with additional EGFR mutation [166]. Other ongoing clinical trials study the potential benefits of combining anti-angiogenic TKIs (e.g., apatinib, endostatin, and anlotinib) with EGFR-TKIs [167].

There are also studies proposing TKI combination with other target inhibitors including monoclonal antibodies. Researches are exploring possibilities of combinations of brigatinib and anti-EGFR antibodies, third-generation TKIs with MEK inhibitors, and osimertinib with oxidative phosphorylation inhibitors etc. [165]. For acute lymphocytic lymphoma, a WEE1 inhibitor AZD-1775 is proven to significantly enhance the efficacy of several tyrosine kinase inhibitors, such as imatinib, bosutinib, and ponatinib [168], or similarly, vitamin K1 with sorafenib in treating HCC [151] and antiestrogen fulvestrant with vandetanib in NSCLC.

Combination approach is promising, yet limited by potential toxicity. Combination of drug effects is true for both positive and side effects. Many studies echoed that concurrent chemotherapy and TKI therapy yielded no added benefits. Therefore, it is important to understand the mechanism of action of the two therapies and understand their interaction, thus design the best administration schedule. Taking TKIs and chemotherapy in an intercalated manner may reduce inhibitory drug interaction. A study compared synchronized administration and intercalated administration of the two therapies [101], and found that intercalated administration schedule improved PFS and OS [169]. More and more studies are thus conducted on the administration schedule and yielded similar results [63].

4.3 Wisdom from traditional Chinese medicine (TCM)

TCM has long been used to treat different cancers and are often shown with clinical efficacy. TCM herbs are able to stabilize tumor growth, control patient symptoms and alleviate side effects, and ultimately improve quality of life of patients [161]. Many researches are thus dedicated to discovering novel drugs by uncovering therapeutic potentials of various natural compounds.

Accumulating studies have been discovering tyrosine kinase inhibiting effects from natural compounds. Many TCM herbs contain natural compounds that are capable of interacting with multiple cellular targets [161]. Various molecules from traditional Chinese medicine are being discovered with tyrosine kinase inhibiting effects and these include 2-O-caffeoyl tartaric acid, emetine, rosmaricine, and 2-O-feruloyl tartaric acid, which are potential EGFR inhibitors [170]. Another meta-analysis identified another 24 kinase inhibitors from TCM [171]. Network pharmacology enables us to discover more of such molecules and their targets [161]. Using natural compounds as drugs is relatively safe and exhibit less side effects [161].

On the other hand, complementary use of TCM has been actively discussed in recent years. Many recent studies have been conducted. They appear to be able to increase efficacy as well as reduce toxicity when combined with TKI therapy [161, 172]. Some studies showed that TCM work synergistically with EGFR-TKI and has additional effect of alleviating TKI induced toxicity [173]. They are able to significantly raise overall response rates, disease control rate, 1-year survival rate, 2-year survival rate, and improvement/stable Karnofsky Performance scores of tumors. Severe toxicity for rash was decreased, so were nausea, vomiting, and diarrhea [174, 175]. The strategy of minimizing or alleviating side effects of TKIs may be potential. This could help increase tolerability of patients and also reduce drug-related adverse events and subsequent possible drug reduction and discontinuation, which will have a toll on TKI therapy effectiveness.

4.4 Improve patient selection

The drug effects of TKIs can be drastically different in two patients. It can work miracles in one, but have no effect at all in another. The genetic makeup of a patient's tumor is a huge predicting value of the efficacy of the TKI. Various studies have shown the correspondence between genetic profiling and therapy response [176, 177]. Thus, it is vital to perform procedures to select the population of patients responsive toward the TKI. In the new era of personalized medicine, the most effective way of using TKIs to treat cancer is to consider each patient/tumor individually and to determine the strategy that specifically targets the consequences of altered genetics of the tumor. Not simply which TKI to use, but also which combination of TKIs and which combination of therapies.

4.5 Repeated monitoring, including repeated biopsy/ liquid biopsy

It was proposed that in order to overcome the limitation of AR in TKIs, repeated tumor biopsies should be done during the course of treatment. This is to give us the ability to spot mutations early and learn its resistance mechanism, thus allowing intervention prior to standard detection of radiographic signs of progression. The specific agent/combination against that particular resistance mechanism can thus be selected.

Yet multiple resistance mechanisms within a single patient, especially between multiple lesions in a patient, pose challenges for biopsy. Besides, biopsies are not accessible for all tumors and are also invasive to the patient. Studies have proposed repeated liquid biopsies as a solution [178]. Liquid biopsy checks for tumor DNA circulating in the blood, which is shed into the bloodstream by tumors all around the body, thus allowing us to peer into the tumor genome in distinct subclones in different metastatic lesions within the patient. It is more effective in learning the heterogeneity and multiple resistance mechanisms than performing a single lesion biopsy. It being less invasive (a simple blood draw will suffice), also allows a more frequent sampling.

4.6 Improve patient compliance

Patient compliance does make a big difference in treatment outcome. Studies have proven that those with higher adherence did achieve better results in achieving CCyR and MMR [113]. Since many TKIs are orally administered, of long-term usage, and in some cases, self-administered in an out-patient setting, patient compliance could pose a serious challenge, especially with irregular drug schedule, such as one with drug holidays. Patient education is one of the ways we could improve patient compliance. Perhaps systems for patient monitoring could also be developed, including system like DOTs therapy for TB patients, where out-patients are required to come to the clinic and take the medicine in front of the healthcare workers and official record is made. Other suggestions include designing phone apps for patients to keep track of their drug schedule.

4.7 Generic drug use

Generic drug use could be a possible solution to high cost of TKIs [179]. Researches on generic versions of various drugs have been conducted [180]. Studies have shown that generic imatinib and Brand named imatinib (Gleevec) showed no difference in efficacy [181]. Aside from imatinib, many TKIs are currently available in generic form, including dasatinib and sorafenib. Yet the quality of generic drugs is not always certified and has to be judged case by case.

4.8 Exploring the potential of TKI therapy termination

Many TKIs are believed to be required to be administered a lifetime. This has posed certain difficulties, including inconvenience to the patients, accumulative side effects, financial burden to the hospital and patient etc. Many studies are thus working on the possibility of discontinuing TKI therapy after a certain response is achieved. Some researches have identified specific subsets of patient populations which could consider discontinuation of TKIs [182].

5. Conclusion

Although TKIs have a very high clinical efficacy upon initial administration, the frequency of acquired resistance is too high, making it not as effective in improving overall survival. There are however many ways we can resort to, in order to prolong the period of stable disease, before progression. These include using multi-targeted approaches, or combination approaches, although it is also accompanied with more severe side effects. Resorting to natural compounds, for example, those from TCM, could be a potential way. They are often multitargeted and not as potent, thus allowing multitarget inhibition without bringing about severe toxicities. Adequate monitoring of disease status and patient adherence is another simple yet effective way to improve the performance of TKIs. Being able to make timely adaptations to treatment plan can play a vital role in prolonging survival. Another direction would be to place more emphasis on patient selection. There are many factors that could help us predict the patient's sensitivity and response toward that TKI. TKI should not be used as an empirical treatment, which would be too cost-ineffective. Even for the same cancer same stage, the specific genetic constitution of each tumor differ from each other, and choice of TKI may vary dependently. Hence, personalized treatment is the key.

Acknowledgements

The study was financially supported by grants from the research council of the University of Hong Kong (Project Codes: 104004092, 104004460, and 104004746), the Research Grants Committee (RGC) of Hong Kong, HKSAR (Project Codes: 764708, 766211, and 17152116), Wong's Donation on Modern Oncology of Chinese Medicine (Project code: 200006276), and Gala Family Trust (Project Code: 200007008).

Author details

Venice Wing Tung Ho, Hor Yue Tan, Ning Wang and Yibin Feng*
School of Chinese Medicine, Li Ka Shing Faculty of Medicine, The University of Hong Kong, Pokfulam, Hong Kong, People's Republic of China

*Address all correspondence to: yfeng@hku.hk

References

[1] Arora A, Scholar EM. Role of tyrosine kinase inhibitors in cancer therapy. Journal of Pharmacology and Experimental Therapeutics. 2005;**315**(3):971-979

[2] Cammack R, et al. Tyrosine Kinase. Oxford, England, UK: Oxford University Press; 2008

[3] Maruyama IN. Mechanisms of activation of receptor tyrosine kinases: Monomers or dimers. Cell. 2014;**3**(2):304-330

[4] Perona R. Cell signalling: Growth factors and tyrosine kinase receptors. Clinical & Translational Oncology. 2006;**8**(2):77-82

[5] Witsch E, Sela M, Yarden Y. Roles for growth factors in cancer progression. Physiology (Bethesda). 2010;**25**(2):85-101

[6] Aaronson S. Growth factors and cancer. Science. 1991;**254**(5035):1146-1153

[7] Goustin AS et al. Growth factors and cancer. 1986;**46**(3):1015-1029

[8] Posner I et al. Kinetics of inhibition by tyrphostins of the tyrosine kinase activity of the epidermal growth factor receptor and analysis by a new computer program. Molecular Pharmacology. 1994;**45**(4):673-683

[9] FDA Approved Drugs for Oncology. 2018. Available from: http://www.centerwatch.com/drug-information/fda-approved-drugs/therapeutic-area/12/oncology

[10] Cismowski MJ. Tyrosine kinase inhibitors. In: Enna SJ, Bylund DB, editors. xPharm: The Comprehensive Pharmacology Reference. New York: Elsevier; 2007. pp. 1-4

[11] Sequist LV. Second-generation epidermal growth factor receptor tyrosine kinase inhibitors in non-small cell lung cancer. The Oncologist. 2007;**12**(3):325-330

[12] Iqbal N, Iqbal N. Imatinib: A breakthrough of targeted therapy in cancer. Chemotherapy Research and Practice. 2014;**2014**:357027

[13] Imatinib-Drugbank. 2018. Available from: https://www.drugbank.ca/drugs/DB00619 [cited: November 2, 2018]

[14] Nowell PC. The minute chromosome (Phl) in chronic granulocytic leukemia. Blut. 1962;**8**:65-66

[15] Sillaber C et al. Chronic myeloid leukemia: Pathophysiology, diagnostic parameters, and current treatment concepts. Wiener Klinische Wochenschrift. 2003;**115**(13-14):485-504

[16] O'Brien SG, Guihot F, Larson RA, Gathmann I, Baccarani M, Cervantes F, et al. Imatinib compared with interferon and low-dose cytarabine for newly diagnosed chronic-phase chronic myeloid leukemia. New England Journal of Medicine. 2003;**348**(11):994-1004

[17] Hughes TP et al. Frequency of major molecular responses to imatinib or interferon alfa plus cytarabine in newly diagnosed chronic myeloid leukemia. The New England Journal of Medicine. 2003;**349**(15):1423-1432

[18] Deininger M et al. International randomized study of interferon vs STI571 (IRIS) 8-year follow up: Sustained survival and low risk for progression or events in patients with newly diagnosed chronic myeloid leukemia in chronic phase (CML-CP) treated with imatinib. Blood. 2009;**114**(22):1126

[19] Deininger M, Buchdunger E, Druker BJ. The development of imatinib as a therapeutic agent for chronic myeloid leukemia. Blood. 2005;**105**(7):2640-2653

[20] Thielen N et al. Preliminary results from a phase III trial of imatinib versus imatinib in combination with cytarabine in patients with first chronic phase myeloid leukemia. Blood. 2011;**118**(21):2758

[21] Guilhot F et al. Significant higher rates of undetectable molecular residual disease and molecular responses with pegylated form of interferon a2a in combination with imatinib (IM) for the treatment of newly diagnosed chronic phase (CP) chronic myeloid leukaemia (CML) patients (pts): Confirmatory results at 18 months of part 1 of the spirit phase III Randomized trial of the French CML Group (FI LMC). Blood. 2009;**114**(22):340

[22] Leis JF et al. Management of life-threatening pulmonary leukostasis with single agent imatinib mesylate during CML myeloid blast crisis. Haematologica. 2004;**89**(9):Ecr30

[23] Sawyers CL et al. Imatinib induces hematologic and cytogenetic responses in patients with chronic myelogenous leukemia in myeloid blast crisis: Results of a phase II study. Blood. 2002;**99**(10):3530-3539

[24] Chauffaille MdLLF et al. Frequency and diversity of variant philadelphia chromosome in chronic myeloid leukemia patients. Blood. 2011;**118**(21):4903

[25] Ujjan ID et al. Cytogenetic and molecular analyses of philadelphia chromosome variants in CML (chronic myeloid leukemia) patients from Sindh using Karyotyping and RT-PCR. Pakistan Journal of Medical Sciences. 2015;**31**(4):936-940

[26] Min KW, Leabu M. Interstitial cells of Cajal (ICC) and gastrointestinal stromal tumor (GIST): Facts, speculations, and myths. Journal of Cellular and Molecular Medicine. 2006;**10**(4):995-1013

[27] Heinrich MC et al. PDGFRA activating mutations in gastro-intestinal stromal tumors. Science. 2003;**299**(5607):708-710

[28] Heinrich MC et al. Kinase mutations and imatinib response in patients with metastatic gastrointestinal stromal tumor. Journal of Clinical Oncology. 2003;**21**(23):4342-4349

[29] Zhao X, Yue C. Gastrointestinal stromal tumor. Journal of Gastro-intestinal Oncology. 2012;**3**(3):189-208

[30] Dematteo RP et al. Adjuvant imatinib mesylate after resection of localised, primary gastrointestinal stromal tumour: A randomised, double-blind, placebo-controlled trial. Lancet. 2009;**373**(9669):1097-1104

[31] Blackstein M. Risk assessment for tumor recurrence after surgical resection of localized primary gastrointestinal stromal tumor (GIST). North American Intergroup Phase III Trial ACOSOG Z9001. ASCO GI Cancer Symposium. 2010;**28** (Suppl 4):6

[32] Duffaud F, Salas S, Huynh T. Recent advances in the management of gastrointestinal stromal tumors. F1000 Medicine Reports. 2010;**2**:36

[33] Ksienski D. Imatinib mesylate: Past successes and future challenges in the treatment of gastrointestinal stromal tumors. Clinical Medicine Insights: Oncology. 2011;**5**:365-379

[34] Van Glabbeke M et al. Initial and late resistance to imatinib in advanced gastrointestinal stromal tumors are predicted by different prognostic

factors: A European Organisation for Research and Treatment of Cancer-Italian Sarcoma Group-Australasian Gastrointestinal Trials Group Study. Journal of Clinical Oncology. 2005;**23**(24):5795-5804

[35] Blanke CD et al. Long-term results from a randomized phase II trial of standard-versus higher-dose imatinib mesylate for patients with unresectable or metastatic gastrointestinal stromal tumors expressing KIT. Journal of Clinical Oncology. 2008;**26**(4):620-625

[36] Blanke CD et al. Phase III randomized, intergroup trial assessing imatinib mesylate at two dose levels in patients with unresectable or metastatic gastrointestinal stromal tumors expressing the kit receptor tyrosine kinase: S0033. Journal of Clinical Oncology. 2008;**26**(4):626-632

[37] Verweij J et al. Progression-free survival in gastrointestinal stromal tumours with high-dose imatinib: Randomised trial. Lancet. 2004;**364**(9440):1127-1134

[38] Schlemmer M et al. Activity and side effects of imatinib in patients with gastrointestinal stromal tumors: Data from a german multicenter trial. European Journal of Medical Research. 2011;**16**(5):206-212

[39] Liu-Dumlao T et al. Philadelphia-positive acute lymphoblastic leukemia: Current treatment options. Current Oncology Reports. 2012;**14**(5):387-394

[40] Yanada M et al. High complete remission rate and promising outcome by combination of imatinib and chemotherapy for newly diagnosed BCR-ABL-positive acute lymphoblastic leukemia: A phase II study by the Japan Adult Leukemia Study Group. Journal of Clinical Oncology. 2006;**24**(3):460-466

[41] Kerob D et al. Imatinib mesylate as a preoperative therapy in dermatofibrosarcoma: Results of a multicenter phase II study on 25 patients. Clinical Cancer Research. 2010;**16**(12):3288-3295

[42] Han A et al. Neoadjuvant imatinib therapy for dermatofibrosarcoma protuberans. Archives of Dermatology. 2009;**145**(7):792-796

[43] Qu S-Q et al. Long-term outcomes of imatinib in patients with FIP1L1/PDGFRA associated chronic eosinophilic leukemia: Experience of a single center in China. Oncotarget. 2016;**7**(22):33229-33236

[44] Alvarez-Twose I et al. Imatinib in systemic mastocytosis: A phase IV clinical trial in patients lacking exon 17 KIT mutations and review of the literature. Oncotarget. 2017;**8**(40):68950-68963

[45] Valent P et al. Long-lasting complete response to imatinib in a patient with systemic mastocytosis exhibiting wild type KIT. American Journal of Blood Research. 2014;**4**(2):93-100

[46] Penel N et al. Imatinib for progressive and recurrent aggressive fibromatosis (desmoid tumors): An FNCLCC/French Sarcoma Group phase II trial with a long-term follow-up. Annals of Oncology. 2011;**22**(2):452-457

[47] Hodi FS et al. Imatinib for melanomas harboring mutationally activated or amplified KIT arising on mucosal, acral, and chronically sun-damaged skin. Journal of Clinical Oncology. 2013;**31**(26):3182-3190

[48] Koon HB et al. Phase II trial of imatinib in AIDS-associated Kaposi's sarcoma: AIDS Malignancy Consortium Protocol 042. Journal of Clinical Oncology. 2014;**32**(5):402-408

[49] Hindi N et al. Imatinib in advanced chordoma: A retrospective case series analysis. European Journal of Cancer. 2015;**51**(17):2609-2614

[50] Casali PG et al. Imatinib mesylate in chordoma. Cancer. 2004;**101**(9):2086-2097

[51] Safra T et al. Weekly paclitaxel with intermittent imatinib mesylate (Gleevec): Tolerance and activity in recurrent epithelial ovarian cancer. Anticancer Research. 2010;**30**(9):3243-3247

[52] Ha HT et al. A phase II study of imatinib in patients with advanced anaplastic thyroid cancer. Thyroid. 2010;**20**(9):975-980

[53] Hensley ML, Ford JM. Imatinib treatment: Specific issues related to safety, fertility, and pregnancy. Seminars in Hematology. 2003;**40**(2 Suppl 2):21-25

[54] Molina JR et al. Non-small cell lung cancer: Epidemiology, risk factors, treatment, and survivorship. Mayo Clinic Proceedings. 2008;**83**(5):584-594

[55] Sebastian M, Schmittel A, Reck M. First-line treatment of EGFR-mutated nonsmall cell lung cancer: Critical review on study methodology. European Respiratory Review. 2014;**23**(131):92-105

[56] Tseng C-H et al. EGFR mutation, smoking, and gender in advanced lung adenocarcinoma. Oncotarget. 2017;**8**(58):98384-98393

[57] Graham RP et al. Worldwide frequency of commonly detected EGFR mutations. Archives of Pathology & Laboratory Medicine. 2018;**142**(2):163-167

[58] Mok TS et al. Gefitinib or carboplatin-paclitaxel in pulmonary adenocarcinoma. The New England Journal of Medicine. 2009;**361**(10):947-957

[59] Maemondo M et al. Gefitinib or chemotherapy for non-small-cell lung cancer with mutated EGFR. The New England Journal of Medicine. 2010;**362**(25):2380-2388

[60] Nakamura A et al. Phase III study comparing gefitinib monotherapy (G) to combination therapy with gefitinib, carboplatin, and pemetrexed (GCP) for untreated patients (pts) with advanced non-small cell lung cancer (NSCLC) with EGFR mutations (NEJ009). Journal of Clinical Oncology. 2018;**36**(15_suppl):9005

[61] Zhou C et al. Erlotinib versus chemotherapy as first-line treatment for patients with advanced EGFR mutation-positive non-small-cell lung cancer (OPTIMAL, CTONG-0802): A multicentre, open-label, randomised, phase 3 study. The Lancet Oncology. 2011;**12**(8):735-742

[62] Wen F et al. OPTIMAL and ENSURE trials-based combined cost-effectiveness analysis of erlotinib versus chemotherapy for the first-line treatment of Asian patients with non-squamous non-small-cell lung cancer. BMJ Open. 2018;**8**(4):e020128

[63] Xu JL et al. Chemotherapy plus erlotinib versus chemotherapy alone for treating advanced non-small cell lung cancer: A meta-analysis. PLoS One. 2015;**10**(7):e0131278

[64] Zhang W et al. Gefitinib provides similar effectiveness and improved safety than erlotinib for east Asian populations with advanced non-small cell lung cancer: A meta-analysis. BMC Cancer. 2018;**18**(1):780

[65] Midha A, Dearden S, McCormack R. EGFR mutation incidence in non-small-cell lung cancer of adenocarcinoma histology: A systematic review and global map by ethnicity (mutMapII). American Journal of Cancer Research. 2015;**5**(9):2892-2911

[66] Lovly C, Horn L, Pao W. Molecular Profiling of Lung Cancer. My Cancer Genome. Nashville, Tennessee: Vanderbilt-Ingram Cancer Center; 2018

[67] Krawczyk P et al. Comparison of the effectiveness of erlotinib, gefitinib, and afatinib for treatment of non-small cell lung cancer in patients with common and rare EGFR gene mutations. Oncology Letters. 2017;**13**(6):4433-4444

[68] Wu JY, Shih JY. Effectiveness of tyrosine kinase inhibitors on uncommon E709X epidermal growth factor receptor mutations in non-small-cell lung cancer. OncoTargets and Therapy. 2016;**9**:6137-6145

[69] Zhou X et al. Gefitinib inhibits the proliferation of pancreatic cancer cells via cell cycle arrest. Anatomical Record (Hoboken, NJ). 2009;**292**(8):1122-1127

[70] Chua DT et al. Phase II study of gefitinib for the treatment of recurrent and metastatic nasopharyngeal carcinoma. Head & Neck. 2008;**30**(7):863-867

[71] Dragovich T et al. Phase II trial of erlotinib in gastroesophageal junction and gastric adenocarcinomas: SWOG 0127. Journal of Clinical Oncology. 2006;**24**(30):4922-4927

[72] Wainberg ZA et al. Phase II trial of modified FOLFOX6 and erlotinib in patients with metastatic or advanced adenocarcinoma of the oesophagus and gastro-oesophageal junction. British Journal of Cancer. 2011;**105**(6):760-765

[73] Schilder RJ et al. A phase II trial of erlotinib in recurrent squamous cell carcinoma of the cervix: A Gynecologic Oncology Group Study. International Journal of Gynecological Cancer. 2009;**19**(5):929-933

[74] Gordon MS et al. Phase II study of erlotinib in patients with locally advanced or metastatic papillary histology renal cell cancer: SWOG S0317. Journal of Clinical Oncology. 2009;**27**(34):5788-5793

[75] Llovet JM, Hernandez-Gea V. Hepatocellular carcinoma: reasons for phase III failure and novel perspectives on trial design. Clinical Cancer Research. 2014;**20**(8):2072-2079

[76] Forsythe B, Faulkner K. Overview of the tolerability of gefitinib (IRESSA) monotherapy: Clinical experience in non-small-cell lung cancer. Drug Safety. 2004;**27**(14):1081-1092

[77] Zhang W et al. Gefitinib provides similar effectiveness and improved safety than erlotinib for advanced non-small cell lung cancer: A meta-analysis. Medicine. 2018;**97**(16):e0460

[78] Ravaud A et al. Real-life patterns of use and effectiveness of sunitinib in patients with metastatic renal cell carcinoma: The SANTORIN study. Journal of Clinical Oncology. 2013;**31**(6_suppl):400

[79] Motzer RJ et al. Overall survival and updated results for sunitinib compared with interferon alfa in patients with metastatic renal cell carcinoma. Journal of Clinical Oncology. 2009;**27**(22):3584-3590

[80] Gore ME et al. Final results from the large sunitinib global expanded-access trial in metastatic renal cell carcinoma. British Journal of Cancer. 2015;**113**(1):12-19

[81] Bellmunt J et al. Phase I study of sunitinib in combination with gemcitabine and capecitabine for first-line treatment of metastatic or unresectable renal cell carcinoma. The Oncologist. 2014;**19**(9):917-918

[82] Schmid TA, Gore ME. Sunitinib in the treatment of metastatic renal cell carcinoma. Therapeutic Advances in Urology. 2016;**8**(6):348-371

[83] Guevremont C et al. Sorafenib in the management of metastatic renal cell carcinoma. Current Oncology. 2009;**16**(Suppl 1):S27-S32

[84] Escudier B et al. Sorafenib in advanced clear-cell renal-cell carcinoma. The New England Journal of Medicine. 2007;**356**(2):125-134

[85] Zhang H-L et al. Sorafenib versus sunitinib as first-line treatment agents in Chinese patients with metastatic renal cell carcinoma: The largest multicenter retrospective analysis of survival and prognostic factors. BMC Cancer. 2017;**17**(1):16

[86] Michel MS et al. SWITCH: A randomized sequential open-label study to evaluate efficacy and safety of sorafenib (SO)/sunitinib (SU) versus SU/SO in the treatment of metastatic renal cell cancer (mRCC). Journal of Clinical Oncology. 2014;**32**(4_suppl):393

[87] Li L et al. The Ras/Raf/MEK/ERK signaling pathway and its role in the occurrence and development of HCC. Oncology Letters. 2016;**12**(5):3045-3050

[88] Zhang L et al. VEGF is essential for the growth and migration of human hepatocellular carcinoma cells. Molecular Biology Reports. 2012;**39**(5):5085-5093

[89] Chaparro M et al. Review article: Pharmacological therapy for hepatocellular carcinoma with sorafenib and other oral agents. Alimentary Pharmacology & Therapeutics. 2008;**28**(11-12):1269-1277

[90] Bruix J et al. Efficacy and safety of sorafenib in patients with advanced hepatocellular carcinoma: Subanalyses of a phase III trial. Journal of Hepatology. 2012;**57**(4):821-829

[91] Llovet JM et al. Sorafenib in advanced hepatocellular carcinoma. The New England Journal of Medicine. 2008;**359**(4):378-390

[92] Abou-Alfa GK et al. Doxorubicin plus sorafenib vs doxorubicin alone in patients with advanced hepatocellular carcinoma: A randomized trial. JAMA. 2010;**304**(19):2154-2160

[93] Sanoff HK et al. Sorafenib Effectiveness in Advanced Hepatocellular Carcinoma. The Oncologist. 2016

[94] Younus J et al. Sunitinib malate for gastrointestinal stromal tumour in imatinib mesylate-resistant patients: Recommendations and evidence. Current Oncology. 2010;**17**(4):4-10

[95] Demetri GD et al. Efficacy and safety of sunitinib in patients with advanced gastrointestinal stromal tumour after failure of imatinib: A randomised controlled trial. Lancet. 2006;**368**(9544):1329-1338

[96] Mulet-Margalef N, Garcia-del-Muro X. Sunitinib in the treatment of gastrointestinal stromal tumor: Patient selection and perspectives. OncoTargets and Therapy. 2016;**9**:7573-7582

[97] Kefeli U et al. Efficacy of sorafenib in patients with gastrointestinal stromal tumors in the third- or fourth-line treatment: A retrospective multicenter experience. Oncology Letters. 2013;**6**(2):605-611

[98] Durante C et al. Long-term outcome of 444 patients with distant metastases from papillary and follicular thyroid carcinoma: Benefits and limits of radioiodine therapy. The Journal of Clinical Endocrinology and Metabolism. 2006;**91**(8):2892-2899

[99] Brose MS et al. Sorafenib in locally advanced or metastatic, radioactive iodine-refractory, differentiated thyroid cancer: A randomized,

double-blind, phase 3 trial. Lancet. 2014;**384**(9940):319-328

[100] van der Veldt AA et al. Predictive factors for severe toxicity of sunitinib in unselected patients with advanced renal cell cancer. British Journal of Cancer. 2008;**99**(2):259-265

[101] Zhang M, Liu M, Wang Y. Clinical efficacy of EGFR-TKIs in combination with chemotherapy in patients with advanced non-small cell lung cancer harboring EGFR mutations. Journal of Thoracic Disease. 2016;**8**(10):E1293-E1295

[102] Di Paolo A et al. Sunitinib in metastatic renal cell carcinoma: The pharmacological basis of the alternative 2/1 schedule. Frontiers in Pharmacology. 2017;**8**:523

[103] Najjar YG et al. A 2 weeks on and 1 week off schedule of sunitinib is associated with decreased toxicity in metastatic renal cell carcinoma. European Journal of Cancer. 2014;**50**(6):1084-1089

[104] Schuette K et al. Tolerability of sorafenib in the treatment of hepatocellular carcinoma (HCC) in patients with Child A and B liver cirrhosis. Journal of Clinical Oncology. 2009;**27**(15S):e15593

[105] Naito S et al. Overall survival and good tolerability of long-term use of sorafenib after cytokine treatment: Final results of a phase II trial of sorafenib in Japanese patients with metastatic renal cell carcinoma. BJU International. 2011;**108**(11):1813-1819

[106] Giles FJ. New directions in the treatment of imatinib failure and/or resistance. Seminars in Hematology. 2009;**46**(2 Suppl 3):S27-S33

[107] Aguilera DG, Tsimberidou AM. Dasatinib in chronic myeloid leukemia: A review. Therapeutics and Clinical Risk Management. 2009;**5**(2):281-289

[108] Shah NP et al. Long-term outcome with dasatinib after imatinib failure in chronic-phase chronic myeloid leukemia: Follow-up of a phase 3 study. Blood. 2014;**123**(15):2317-2324

[109] Hochhaus A et al. Dasatinib induces durable cytogenetic responses in patients with chronic myelogenous leukemia in chronic phase with resistance or intolerance to imatinib. Leukemia. 2008;**22**(6):1200-1206

[110] Kantarjian H et al. Dasatinib versus imatinib in newly diagnosed chronic-phase chronic myeloid leukemia. The New England Journal of Medicine. 2010;**362**(24):2260-2270

[111] Kantarjian H et al. Nilotinib in imatinib-resistant CML and Philadelphia chromosome–positive ALL. The New England Journal of Medicine. 2006;**354**(24):2542-2551

[112] Saglio G et al. Nilotinib versus imatinib for newly diagnosed chronic myeloid leukemia. The New England Journal of Medicine. 2010;**362**(24):2251-2259

[113] Di Bella NJ et al. The effectiveness of tyrosine kinase inhibitors and molecular monitoring patterns in newly diagnosed patients with chronic myeloid leukemia in the community setting. Clinical Lymphoma, Myeloma & Leukemia. 2015;**15**(10):599-605

[114] Cortes JE et al. Bosutinib versus imatinib for newly diagnosed chronic myeloid leukemia: Results from the randomized BFORE trial. Journal of Clinical Oncology. 2018;**36**(3):231-237

[115] Kwak J-Y et al. Efficacy and safety of radotinib compared with imatinib in newly diagnosed chronic phase chronic myeloid leukemia patients: 12 months result of phase 3 clinical trial. Blood. 2015;**126**(23):476

[116] Adverse Reactions. Pfitzer Canada Inc. 2018. https://www.pfizermedicalinformation.ca/en-ca/bosulif/adverse-reactions

[117] Sullivan I, Planchard D. Next-generation EGFR tyrosine kinase inhibitors for treating EGFR-mutant lung cancer beyond first line. Frontiers in Medicine. 2016;**3**:76

[118] Sequist LV et al. Phase III study of afatinib or cisplatin plus pemetrexed in patients with metastatic lung adenocarcinoma with EGFR mutations. Journal of Clinical Oncology. 2013;**31**(27):3327-3334

[119] Wu YL et al. Dacomitinib versus gefitinib as first-line treatment for patients with EGFR-mutation-positive non-small-cell lung cancer (ARCHER 1050): A randomised, open-label, phase 3 trial. The Lancet Oncology. 2017;**18**(11):1454-1466

[120] Reckamp KL et al. A phase 2 trial of dacomitinib (PF-00299804), an oral, irreversible pan-HER (human epidermal growth factor receptor) inhibitor, in patients with advanced non-small cell lung cancer after failure of prior chemotherapy and erlotinib. Cancer. 2014;**120**(8):1145-1154

[121] Sternberg CN et al. Pazopanib in locally advanced or metastatic renal cell carcinoma: Results of a randomized phase III trial. Journal of Clinical Oncology. 2010;**28**(6):1061-1068

[122] van Geel RMJM, Beijnen JH, Schellens JHM. Concise drug review: Pazopanib and axitinib. The Oncologist. 2012;**17**(8):1081-1089

[123] Pazopanib outscores sunitinib on tolerability. Cancer Discovery. 2014;**4**(1):Of8. http://cancerdiscovery.aacrjournals.org/content/4/1/OF8, https://www.ncbi.nlm.nih.gov/pubmed/24402960

[124] Motzer RJ et al. Tivozanib versus sorafenib as initial targeted therapy for patients with metastatic renal cell carcinoma: Results from a phase III trial. Journal of Clinical Oncology. 2013;**31**(30):3791-3799

[125] Motzer RJ. AVEO and Astellas Announce Positive Findings from TIVO-1 Superiority Study of Tivozanib in First Line Advanced RCC. Astellas. 2012. https://newsroom.astellas.us/news-releases?item=136985

[126] Grothey A et al. Regorafenib monotherapy for previously treated metastatic colorectal cancer (CORRECT): An international, multicentre, randomised, placebo-controlled, phase 3 trial. The Lancet. 2013;**381**(9863):303-312

[127] Demetri GD et al. Efficacy and safety of regorafenib for advanced gastrointestinal stromal tumours after failure of imatinib and sunitinib (GRID): An international, multicentre, randomised, placebo-controlled, phase 3 trial. The Lancet. 2013;**381**(9863):295-302

[128] Cortes JE et al. Ponatinib efficacy and safety in Philadelphia chromosome-positive leukemia: Final 5-year results of the phase 2 PACE trial. Blood. 2018;**132**(4):393-404

[129] Soria J-C et al. Osimertinib in untreated EGFR-mutated advanced non-small-cell lung cancer. The New England Journal of Medicine. 2018;**378**(2):113-125

[130] Hsia T-C et al. Comparative effectiveness of concurrent chemoradiotherapy versus EGFR-tyrosine kinase inhibitors for the treatment of clinical stage IIIb lung adenocarcinoma patients with mutant EGFR. Thoracic Cancer. 2018;**9**:1398-1405

[131] Wu L et al. Clinical efficacy of second-generation tyrosine kinase

inhibitors in imatinib-resistant gastrointestinal stromal tumors: A meta-analysis of recent clinical trials. Drug Design, Development and Therapy. 2014;**8**:2061-2067

[132] Ferrari SM et al. Lenvatinib in the therapy of aggressive thyroid cancer: State of the art and new perspectives with patents recently applied. Recent Patents on Anti-Cancer Drug Discovery. 2018;**13**(2):201-208

[133] Archer K. What factors are predictive of survival in patients with non-small-cell lung cancer treated with gefitinib? Thorax. 2007;**62**(9):757

[134] Bonomi PD, Buckingham L, Coon J. Selecting patients for treatment with epidermal growth factor tyrosine kinase inhibitors. Clinical Cancer Research. 2007;**13**(15):4606s-4612s

[135] Stasi I, Cappuzzo F. Second generation tyrosine kinase inhibitors for the treatment of metastatic non-small-cell lung cancer. Translational Respiratory Medicine. 2014;**2**:2

[136] Hirsh V et al. A personalized approach to treatment: Use of egfr tyrosine kinase inhibitors for the treatment of non-small-cell lung cancer in Canada. Journal of Current Oncology. 2012;**19**(2):13

[137] Milojkovic D, Apperley J. Mechanisms of resistance to imatinib and second-generation tyrosine inhibitors in chronic myeloid leukemia. Clinical Cancer Research. 2009;**15**(24):7519-7527

[138] Bixby D, Talpaz M. Mechanisms of resistance to tyrosine kinase inhibitors in chronic myeloid leukemia and recent therapeutic strategies to overcome resistance. ASH Education Program Book. 2009;**2009**(1):461-476

[139] Chen Y-f, Fu L-w. Mechanisms of acquired resistance to tyrosine kinase inhibitors. Acta Pharmaceutica Sinica B. 2011;**1**(4):197-207

[140] Burke AC, Swords RT, Kelly K, Giles FJ. Current status of agents active against the T315I chronic myeloid leukemia phenotype. Expert Opinion on Emerging Drugs. 2011;**16**(1):85-103

[141] Tudor RA et al. Beyond disease-progression: Clinical outcomes after EGFR-TKIs in a cohort of EGFR mutated NSCLC patients. PLoS One. 2017;**12**(8):e0181867

[142] Logue JS, Morrison DK. Complexity in the signaling network: Insights from the use of targeted inhibitors in cancer therapy. Genes & Development. 2012;**26**(7):641-650

[143] Lavi O. Redundancy: A critical obstacle to improving cancer therapy. Cancer Research. 2015;**75**(5):808-812

[144] Parikh AA, Ellis LM. The vascular endothelial growth factor family and its receptors. Hematology/Oncology Clinics of North America. 2004;**18**(5):951-971, vii

[145] Potapova O et al. Contribution of individual targets to the antitumor efficacy of the multitargeted receptor tyrosine kinase inhibitor SU11248. Molecular Cancer Therapeutics. 2006;**5**(5):1280-1289

[146] Morris LG et al. Pan-cancer analysis of intratumor heterogeneity as a prognostic determinant of survival. Oncotarget. 2016;7(9):10051-10063

[147] Paez JG et al. EGFR mutations in lung cancer: Correlation with clinical response to gefitinib therapy. Science. 2004;**304**(5676):1497-1500

[148] Sequist LV et al. Neratinib, an irreversible pan-ErbB receptor tyrosine kinase inhibitor: Results of a phase II trial in patients with advanced non-small-cell lung

cancer. Journal of Clinical Oncology. 2010;**28**(18):3076-3083

[149] Perez-Soler R. The role of erlotinib (Tarceva, OSI 774) in the treatment of non-small cell lung cancer. Clinical Cancer Research. 2004;**10**(12 Pt 2): 4238s-4240s

[150] Hartmann JT et al. Tyrosine kinase inhibitors—A review on pharmacology, metabolism and side effects. Current Drug Metabolism. 2009;**10**(5):470-481

[151] Aravalli RN, Cressman ENK, Steer CJJAoT. Cellular and molecular mechanisms of hepatocellular carcinoma: An update. Archives of Toxicology. 2013;**87**(2):227-247

[152] Padula WV et al. Cost-effectiveness of tyrosine kinase inhibitor treatment strategies for chronic myeloid leukemia in chronic phase after generic entry of imatinib in the United States. JNCI - Journal of the National Cancer Institute. 2016;**108**(7):djw003

[153] Winn AN, Keating NL, Dusetzina SB. Factors associated with tyrosine kinase inhibitor initiation and adherence among medicare beneficiaries with chronic myeloid leukemia. Journal of Clinical Oncology. 2016;**34**(36):4323-4328

[154] Islamagic E et al. The efficacy of generic imatinib as first- and second-line therapy: 3-year follow-up of patients with chronic myeloid leukemia. Clinical Lymphoma, Myeloma & Leukemia. 2017;**17**(4):238-240

[155] Soria JC et al. Gefitinib plus chemotherapy versus placebo plus chemotherapy in EGFR-mutation-positive non-small-cell lung cancer after progression on first-line gefitinib (IMPRESS): A phase 3 randomised trial. The Lancet Oncology. 2015;**16**(8):990-998

[156] Antonescu CR et al. Acquired resistance to imatinib in gastrointestinal stromal tumor occurs through secondary gene mutation. 2005;**11**(11):4182-4190

[157] Péter Csermely VÁ, Pongor S. The efficiency of multi-target drugs: The network approach might help drug design. Trends in Pharmacological Sciences. 2005;**26**(4):178-182

[158] Broekman F, Giovannetti E, Peters GJ. Tyrosine kinase inhibitors: Multi-targeted or single-targeted? World Journal of Clinical Oncology. 2011;**2**(2):80-93

[159] Petrelli A, Giordano S. From single- to multi-target drugs in cancer therapy: When aspecificity becomes an advantage. Current Medicinal Chemistry. 2008;**15**(5):422-432

[160] Medina-Franco JL et al. Shifting from the single to the multitarget paradigm in drug discovery. Drug Discovery Today. 2013;**18**(9-10):495-501

[161] Phani Krishna P, Khajapeer KV, Balakrishnan AP, Rajasekaran B. Multi-Targeted Approach to Treat Drug Resistant CML Using Natural Compounds: A Double Edged Sword. New York, USA: Crimson Publishers; 2018

[162] Johnson DB et al. Acquired BRAF inhibitor resistance: A multicenter meta-analysis of the spectrum and frequencies, clinical behaviour, and phenotypic associations of resistance mechanisms. European Journal of Cancer. 2015;**51**(18):2792-2799

[163] O'Dwyer M. First-line treatment of chronic myeloid leukaemia. Therapeutic Advances in Hematology. 2010;**1**(1):15-22

[164] Zhang S et al. Icotinib enhances lung cancer cell radiosensitivity in vitro and in vivo by inhibiting MAPK/ERK and AKT activation. Clinical

and Experimental Pharmacology & Physiology. 2018;**45**(9):969-977

[165] Tan CS et al. Third generation EGFR TKIs: Current data and future directions. Molecular Cancer. 2018;**17**(1):29

[166] Yamaguchi N et al. Dual ALK and EGFR inhibition targets a mechanism of acquired resistance to the tyrosine kinase inhibitor crizotinib in ALK rearranged lung cancer. Lung Cancer (Amsterdam, Netherlands). 2014;**83**(1):37-43

[167] ClinicalTrials.gov, Zhengtang Chen. Xinqiao Hospital of Chongqing-Identifier: NCT03461185. Anti-Angiogenesis Combine With EGFR-TKI in Advanced Non-Squamous Non Small Cell Lung Cancer. 2018. Available from: https://clinicaltrials.gov/ct2/show/NCT03461185

[168] Ghelli Luserna Di Rora A et al. Targeting WEE1 to enhance conventional therapies for acute lymphoblastic leukemia. Journal of Hematology & Oncology. 2018;**11**(1):99

[169] Wu YL et al. Intercalated combination of chemotherapy and erlotinib for patients with advanced stage non-small-cell lung cancer (FASTACT-2): A randomised, double-blind trial. The Lancet Oncology. 2013;**14**(8):777-786

[170] Yang S-C et al. Identification of potent EGFR inhibitors from TCM Database@Taiwan. PLoS Computational Biology. 2011;7(10):e1002189

[171] Liu M et al. Development of certain protein kinase inhibitors with the components from traditional Chinese medicine. Frontiers in Pharmacology. 2016;7:523

[172] Hu X-Q et al. Advances in synergistic combinations of Chinese herbal medicine for the treatment of cancer. Current Cancer Drug Targets. 2016;**16**(4):346-356

[173] Hung H-Y et al. The efficacy of traditional Chinese herbal medicine in the treatment of EGFR mutated stage IV pulmonary adenocarcinoma patients who received first-line EGFR-TKI treatment. Integrative Cancer Therapies. 2017;**16**(1):126-131

[174] He W, Cheng M. Meta-analysis on effectiveness and safety of traditional Chinese medicine combined with first-generation EGFR-TKI in treating advanced non-small cell lung cancer. Zhongguo Zhong Yao Za Zhi. 2017;**42**(13):2591-2598

[175] Liu ZL et al. Traditional Chinese medicinal herbs combined with epidermal growth factor receptor tyrosine kinase inhibitor for advanced non-small cell lung cancer: A systematic review and meta-analysis. Journal of Integrative Medicine. 2014;**12**(4):346-358

[176] Farber NJ et al. Renal cell carcinoma: The search for a reliable biomarker. Translational Cancer Research. 2017;**6**(3):620-632

[177] Manley BJ, Hakimi AA. Molecular profiling of renal cell carcinoma: Building a bridge towards clinical impact. Current Opinion in Urology. 2016;**26**(5):383-387

[178] Ahronian LG, Corcoran RBJGM. Strategies for monitoring and combating resistance to combination kinase inhibitors for cancer therapy. Genome Medicine. 2017;**9**(1):37

[179] Chen CT, Kesselheim AS. Journey of generic imatinib: A case study in oncology drug pricing. Journal of Oncology Practice. 2017;**13**(6):352-355

[180] Klil-Drori AJ et al. Comparative effectiveness of generic imatinib and

brand-name imatinib for the treatment of chronic myeloid leukemia. Blood. 2015;**126**(23):2778

[181] Kozaric AK et al. The comparison of efficacy between generic and branded imatinib in achievement of overall survival and cytogenetic responses in CML patients in Bosnia and Herzegovina. Blood. 2016;**128**(22):5451

[182] Dvorak P, Lysak D, Vokurka S. Discontinuation of tyrosine kinase inhibitors in chronic myeloid leukemia patients—Worldwide battlefield. Neoplasma. 2015;**62**(2):167-171